AUTHOR'S NOTE

Have you ever wondered how queer couples become parents? If you're straight, probably not. If you're queer, then possibly. Maybe you had a quick Google and struggled to find anything legit. Maybe you learnt a bit but felt overwhelmed by the medical jargon and legal requirements essential to queer parenting. Maybe it was a little too complicated, so you closed your laptop, vowing to revisit it the next day (you didn't).

If you're a lesbian, you could ask your ex-girlfriend. She's now married with two kids, and they all live in Eastbourne because Brighton is too expensive. It might sound like a weird thing to do, asking your ex, but it's not. It's just very lesbian. The more awkward and inappropriate the better! Your ex gives you some information, but it doesn't clarify all that much, and you still don't know where to start because the law seems to have changed again. The law changes all the time! It also cost them £15,000. You don't have £15,000! Does anyone have £15,000 spare?

You consider adoption. Your mate tells you about their gay friends who adopted a five-year-old boy. They were on the waiting list for six years. They had to own their own house. They also needed to have more than one bedroom. I have one bedroom and a living room people sometimes sleep in… does that count?

I work with a trans woman who hopes to have children in the future. When asked about her options, she expresses uncertainty, assuming that her chances are limited due to the lack of information on trans parenting and insufficient access to trans-inclusive healthcare. You think, fuck, she's right. There's not much out there at all. Her friend, a trans man, has the same problem.

The person at the coffee shop around the corner, who is nonbinary, mentioned that because the United Kingdom doesn't legally recognise nonbinary individuals, having children can not only be more complicated but also terrifying when it comes to custody matters. They specifically brought up birth certificates – fucking birth certificates. We'll get to those later.

Remember sex education at school? On one hand, I'm lucky that I was taught anything at all. But on the

A Short History of

QUEER PARENTING

Also by Kirsty Loehr

A Short History of Queer Women

A Short History of

QUEER PARENTING

Including my own...

KIRSTY LOEHR

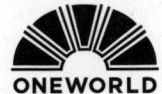

ONEWORLD

A Oneworld Book

First published by Oneworld Publications Ltd in 2025

Copyright © Kirsty Loehr, 2025

ISBN 978-1-83643-080-3
eISBN 978-1-83643-081-0

Typeset by Geethik Technologies
Illustration from *Heather Has Two Mommies* © Diana Souza
Printed and bound in Great Britain by Clays Ltd, Elcograf S.p.A.

The authorised representative in the EEA is eucomply OÜ,
Pärnu mnt 139b–14, 11317 Tallinn, Estonia
(email: hello@eucompliancepartner.com / phone: +33757690241)

Oneworld Publications
10 Bloomsbury Street
London WC1B 3SR
England

For all the queer parents who have come before and those who continue to shape our world – and of course, for Hammy, who changed my life more than I ever thought possible, my closest thing to magic.

And my catties, Max and Mitch, and our dearly missed Marmie (RIP). Pets are also a valid part of a queer person's parental journey, and it's important to honour them whenever we can.

CONTENTS

other hand, the information didn't mean anything to me. It was sex education for heterosexuals – Hi, Section 28! There was a man and a woman. They had sex (almost always in missionary) and then *painlessly* a baby appeared nine months later. They didn't need to be married; they didn't need to have £15,000; and they didn't have to have more than one bedroom. They all fucking smoked and they all fucking drank. Nobody got involved, nobody cared, and nobody asked questions about their gender identity, sexual preferences, salary or ten-year plan.

Heterosexual people have options. They have more direct access to fertility treatments, adoption, fostering and surrogacy. Sure, it's complicated, but it's available, and they also have extra help in terms of funding. There are websites, leaflets, consultations and referrals. The whole system is designed for heterosexual people to reproduce, make more children and live 'normal', respectable lives. Queer people are not invited.

This book is for queer people who have convinced themselves that they don't want children because they were never allowed to think that it might be possible. It's for queer people who thought queer parenting was not an option because it did not exist in history, except that it did... It's also for queer people who *do* know that children are an option but *don't* know where to start.

As with my first book, *A Short History of Queer Women*, I want to both explore and subvert this sensitive subject. It is a subject that can be triggering. I'll look at how queer parenting has developed over the years, and all the different methods involved: inheriting through relationships, co-parenting, adoption, foster care, donor insemination, reciprocal IVF, surrogacy and having children with someone who then becomes an ex (as in what happened to me).

This is a subject that can be inaccessible due to unreliable information on the internet, academic jargon and off-putting legal requirements. I hope that my approach will make a fraught subject more welcoming, enlightening and maybe even funny. I hope that it will give queer people the tools to start their journey, but also the quiet confidence that queer parenting is not a newfangled innovation but something that has been a part of society forever. You are not alone in wanting to start a family. We've been doing this for ages!

A Short History of Queer Women was not an academic history, but a retelling. It was a starting point and, hopefully, an enjoyable one. By the same token, this is not a medical book. I am not an expert on queer parenting – just ask my son. Nor am I an expert on IVF – but I went through it and it was hard, emotional and expensive. Now I am lucky enough to write about it.

LET'S MAKE IT QUEER

Society says that queer parenting is a modern concept, alongside fitness trackers, adult colouring books and air fryers. It's not. Queer parenting can actually be traced as far back as, well, human existence.

A long time ago, a really long time ago, between 14,000 and 40,000 years ago, everybody was shagging everybody, all holes were goals, and days were spent drawing pictures in caves. Hmm, this seems familiar…

My theory goes as follows. Before agriculture, before farming, there were hunter/gatherers and nobody cared what they did with their genitals, nobody cared where they put them, and the concept of gender, relationships and sexuality didn't exist. Before the patriarchy introduced heteronormativity and the world became beige, everyone was just happy *being*. No capitalists, no fragile masculinity, no weird gender role models. Folk just wandered around grunting at one another, killing large cows and starting fires.

Family as a unit certainly didn't exist. Mothers, fathers, wicked stepmothers, creepy fathers-in-law – all these things were yet to come. Parental roles had no place in society and mother-in-law jokes were a delight of the future…

Then things changed. Societal roles shifted. Gender and sexuality became fixed, and the Romans started making jokes about women in the kitchen and, of course, irritating mothers-in-law.

'While your mother-in-law still lives, domestic harmony is out of the question,' writes Decimus Junius Juvenalis (better known as Juvenal) to the knee-slap of his mates and the eye-roll of many a Roman woman.

The word 'family' comes from the Latin word *famulus* or 'servant'… which makes total sense to me now that I'm a mother. But what exactly do we mean by 'family' or even 'parent'?

According to the *Oxford English Dictionary*, a family is a group of people consisting of one set of parents and their children, whether living together or not. A parent is a person who is one of the pro-genitors of a child; a father or mother, a woman or man who takes on parental responsibilities…

If you're like me and had to look up the meaning of 'progenitor', you now know that this means the person you are descended from. Thus, a parent is either an ancestor or someone who takes on parental responsibilities.

Those responsibilities often include:

1   pretending to like other parents
2   pretending to like other children
3   watching *Bluey* (no complaints here, even if the dad does make me feel like a piece of shit with no imagination)

But what's crucial here is that the words 'father' and 'mother', 'woman' and 'man' are used quite prominently when attempting to understand and define what a parental figure might be. In other words, anything that steps outside of that binary is not *really* a parent... but we'll get to that bit later.

For now, let's go further back.

Keep it in the family

Believe it or not, the ancient world was reasonably diverse. I use the words 'reasonably' and 'diverse' cautiously, but it was certainly as varied as Kristen Stewart's relationship history. Sometimes things were boring, and sometimes they were fun. Sometimes it was Robert Pattinson, and sometimes it was Stella Maxwell.

Take the Amazons, hailed by the Greeks as the most powerful women ever – clearly, they'd never witnessed a straight woman's hen night when 'Man! I Feel Like a Woman!' drops. That's true power right there.

The Amazons were the original radical feminists, rebelling against male-dominated societies and setting up camp far away from men. While male historians often doubt their existence, or at least dumb them down, we know they were real because the Greeks wrote about them and everything the Greeks say is true. They never make anything up.

But we do know that this nation of warrior women (who allegedly chopped off their right tit to shoot arrows better) lived without men, only seeking them out once a year to conceive daughters. If they had sons, which, um, was just as likely? Well, they either gave them away or… killed them. FFS, I was rooting for these titless warriors!

The Greeks had been doing 'family' long before the Romans. In Ancient Greece, women were… drum roll… irrelevant. If a family had a daughter but no son, special measures would be put in place to ensure the survival of the family. These measures included marrying the daughter to a male relative so that the daughter's father could adopt him as his son. The father could even adopt his daughter's son if he wanted. It's all very Battersea Dogs Home, isn't it? The phrase 'adopt don't shop' comes to mind.

Over in Egypt, brothers and sisters (usually high-born) would often marry. They would then shack up in a big house as husband and wife, with all their children (nephews and nieces?). One famous example is Cleopatra, who successively married *both* of her younger brothers, Ptolemy XIII and Ptolemy XIV. The marriages weren't great, though, and both ended with her reigning alone, thus disproving the old adage that incest is best.

Then we have various ancient Hindu medical texts portraying the sexual unions of two women, mostly in the context of co-wives. In many of these texts the result is a child, as in the two women conceive. Sometimes a poet will pick up that theme and run with it: for instance, in a fifteenth-century retelling of the birth of King Bhagiratha, 'the two wives of Dilipa took a bath. The young women lived together in extreme love… Both of them knew one another's intentions and enjoyed love play, and one of them conceived.'

If only!

In another version, their son Bhagiratha is 'born of mutual enjoyment between two vaginas' – sadly, this wasn't the case for me, but interesting nonetheless. (Later writers also claimed his very name pays respect to the vulva, or *bhaga*.) And while many of these texts aren't exactly positive accounts (most of the babies end up as misshapen lumps of flesh), the concept of same-sex parenting and producing children is *there*.

In Ancient China, families were led by Confucian moral values in their ancestral worship. This demanded absolute obedience from younger members of the family towards elders, and supposedly resulted in a peaceful and serene lifestyle. I'm listening. But then breastfeeding your sickly mother-in-law was also expected. Earmuffs!

It was also all about the men (when isn't it?) to the point where the most distant male relative was considered more important than the nearest female relative. So like a male cousin of mine, a million times removed, would have more rights over my father's money than, well, me. And if a family had no distant male relatives? Then someone with the same surname would make do, as this was evidence that, at some point in their life, they shared an ancestor. I hope you've taken your antidepressants today!

OK, by now you're probably thinking, 'Where are the gays?' And you're not wrong, it certainly seems that way. Historically, children have been raised in all sorts of ways, and by expanding our definition of 'queer', any family that isn't the usual mum, dad, two kids, dog and cat could technically be considered a 'queer' family – queer doesn't always have to refer to a sexuality, after all. So, by this logic, the concept of queer parenting isn't new in the slightest. But honestly, that's a bit boring – and I wanted to find actual queers, not loopholes! So, as with all of history, if you dig deep enough, you'll find us. We're here, we're queer and we're ready to parent!

Let's begin with China's *Jinglanhui* (the Golden Orchid Society), formed in around 1644, a place where women would go to actively avoid men, like a women's football game, therapy or the bath.

In the Golden Orchid Society, women could not only marry each other, but they could also adopt a daughter together. Oddly the latter was more acceptable than the former. Confusing!

The adopted daughter would then be able to inherit property from her parents. Her parents as in her mother and her other mother... yes, you read that correctly. A leg up on the property ladder plus having *another* mother!

What's funny is that ancient civilisations and queer parenting have a lot more in common than your school curriculum, history books, and modern life would have you believe. Much like pre-colonised Africa. In many ancient African kingdoms, gendered clothes weren't really a thing, as in people wore whatever they fucking wanted. Plus, there were (and still are) several African languages that characterise(d) queerness positively and lovingly.

And then there's the classic proverb, 'It takes a village to raise a child' – often linked to African cultures (although we still don't know for sure where it originated), emphasising the idea that parenting isn't a one- or two-person job, but more of a group project where everyone, from the grandparents to the next-door neighbour, gets involved. This rings especially true for a lot of queer people today who embrace co-parenting, making it a popular choice as they embark on their parenting journeys. (But more on that later… it's a vibe.)

You could say that this 'it takes a village' mentality was weakened when the Europeans decided to colonise the continent and savagely force their own backward shit onto several of these kingdoms. You could also say that this should be remembered when we disparage countries like Uganda or Nigeria for their lack of LGBTQIA+ rights. It wasn't always like that… at least not until the Europeans arrived.

Heading into the Middle Ages, into Southern and Eastern Europe, it was common to see multiple generations of one family all living under one roof. Much like how Gen Z live now but with fourteen unrelated roommates, and the constant anxiety that someone will steal your kombucha from the fridge.

Northern Europeans had other ideas and left the family home as soon as they were married. In fact, many Northern European women never married at all, and we know what that means... THEY WERE ALL LESBIANS. Joke. Not all of them.

But before the Romans, before pre-colonised Africa, before the Golden Orchid Society, there was Sappho. Ah, Sappho, the original lesbian. Soooo lesbian that she invented the guitar pick so she could bang more women. Soooo lesbian that her tragic poetry inspired future dykey writers to come up with even more tragic and depressing songs – cooee, Billie Eilish! Not only was she the original lesbian, but she was also... wait for it... probably the first lesbian parent (that we know of anyway). How exciting!

Yes, according to some (probably lesbian) historians, Sappho supposedly had a daughter named Cleis, which for some reason sounds like a name a lesbian would give to their child. Don't ask me why.

If there was a Cleis, biology would suggest that there was a father of Cleis, but nobody knows (cares) about him, at least Sappho didn't care enough to write about him anyway. Even though that is literally what Sappho did – she wrote about her lovers. That was like her *whole thing*!

Jesus had two dads, and he turned out just fine...

Then we've got the little-known historical figure Jesus Christ.

Brace yourselves (or maybe I should).

The story goes that the 'saviour of the modern world' Jesus Christ had two dads, Joseph and God. And while LGBTQIA+ Christians love this little anecdote, I'm pretty sure non-LGBTQIA+ Christians don't. So, let's make this snappy.

It's quite simple really. Mary was the mother of Jesus. Joseph was the father of Jesus. God was *also* the father of Jesus, you know, like his *other* dad (insert those large emoji eyes). What does this tell us about the rapport between God and Joseph? Who knows! And what about that other Joseph, the one who loved to wear an 'amazing Technicolor dreamcoat'? He also seemed pretty gay to me. Maybe it's a Joseph thing. Hey, my dad is called Joseph and apparently being gay is genetic... but I digress. What we *do* know is that Jesus turned out fine and was actually really sound.

The history of queer parenting is not merely a history of same-sex parents. It's not just two queer people getting together and deciding to have a baby. It's much more than that. It's people challenging heteronormativity in a world that makes it difficult for queer people to live in. And, as we move into the modern age, this becomes much more apparent.

Forging families

What's the first thing you think of when you think of Oscar Wilde? His sharp wit and love for the drama, obvs. If he were alive today, he'd have been live-tweeting the Rebecca Vardy vs Coleen Rooney saga – I mean, he basically invented the celebrity court case. He was also famously gay and went to prison for it. It's what I immediately think about when I think of him. Most queer people do! We do because it was a pivotal point in our history, proving that nobody was safe, not even the rich and famous. But for real, Oscar Wilde, arguably one of the best-known queer figures in Western history, was married to a cis woman and had two kids. A real plot twist for the ages!

Then you've got the self-described sapphist, gardener and top shagger Vita Sackville-West. Vita was married to the bisexual politician Harold Nicolson, a marriage that produced two children. Both Vita and Harold had affairs and relationships outside their marriage and both of their children were aware of these. Their youngest son, Nigel Nicolson, even wrote a book (*Portrait of a*

Marriage) about them that almost proudly detailed their extramarital affairs. I recently had the pleasure of meeting Juliet Nicolson, Vita Sackville-West's granddaughter, and I'd never want to take anything away from Juliet – she's an incredible author in her own right – but, as someone who's completely obsessed with her grandmother, when I met Juliet it felt like I was meeting Vita. It was surreal. I'm also well aware this has absolutely nothing to do with this book, but it was Vita Sackville-West's granddaughter! Sapphic blood! I also wanted to show off.

But anyway, let's talk about the writer Walter Sholto Douglas. Walter, who was assigned female at birth in 1790, presented as a man (in fact many different men) for most of his life. Walter's partner, Isabella Robinson, became pregnant by another man, so to help cover the pregnancy's illegitimacy, Walter married Isabella and took on the role of father.

After the baby was born, Walter and Isabella escaped to Paris under false passports assisted by their mate, Mary Shelley (yes, that one). Imagine your 'mate' being Mary Shelley, and while we're on that topic… Everything that I read about Mary Shelley is cool – her mother was cool, her writing was cool, *she* was cool – but I'll never understand why on earth she married that drip Percy Bysshe

Shelley. And she didn't just marry him, she was like proper in love with him. Seriously, can someone enlighten me? Why? I'd honestly respect her more if she had married Byron; at least he had a bit of flair, even if he was a misogynist wanker, incomprehensible poet and an unforgivable human being. Should I be footnoting these opinions?

So queer people like Oscar Wilde, Vita Sackville-West and Walter Sholto Douglas have been forging families for centuries, figuring out how to exist under the guise of conventional heterosexuality.

They existed, and their families were legitimate. And it wasn't just the intelligentsia. Everyday dummies were doing the same thing. Even working-class queer people were attempting to be their authentic selves while outwardly adhering to what society expected from them.

The Caravan Club (London's greatest bohemian rendezvous, opened in 1934) was a place where men hooked up with men, women hooked up with women, men dressed like women and women dressed like men. It was great until some straight people got wind and called the police. God forbid we have any fun. The papers later described the Caravan as 'an absolute sink of iniquity… frequented by sexual perverts, lesbians and sodomites' – a description that in my eyes is akin to ★ ★ ★ ★ ★ *Guardian*.

After more and more complaints, the police decided to enter the club undercover; you know, to see exactly what was going on in there. It took them a good couple of hours before they revealed themselves to the punters. A couple of hours? How long does it take to spot queer people being queer? All of five seconds in my experience.

When the police finally revealed themselves, several people were arrested and the club was closed down. Then, a few weeks later, in a hotel bedroom, a letter was found. It was written by Cyril Coeur de Leon to the Caravan Club owner, Billy Reynolds.

> *My Dear Billy,*
> *Just a note to say that I am very disappointed about you, I honestly thought that you were queer, but different from the others, and I liked you very much. I didn't intend coming to the Club last night only I felt that I must see you. I have only been queer since I came to London about two years ago, before then I knew nothing about it, as I told you I am married and have a little girl two years of age, and I still like girls occasionally, there are very few boys with whom I want to have an affair with, I like them all as friends but nothing more. I have a boy staying with me*

and who is really my affair, we have been together now since I came to town and I like him very much, and I think he is a better pal to me than any woman could ever be, altho' sometimes I wish that I was still normal as queer people are very temperamental and dissatisfied. I honestly hoped to have an affair with you Billy, and I shall only come to the Club to see you. Well it is now 10 p.m. and I have just got up out of bed so must close down and have a bath and dress, and hope that you will excuse my telling you all this only as I say, I like you very very much and feel that I can talk this way to you. Please be a dear boy and destroy this note, and do not mention it to anyone as this is just between you and I. I shall look forward to seeing you in about a couple of hours. Until then.

Your Very Sincere friend always,
Cyril Coeur de Leon[1]

Look, the cheating on your wife who is at home with your daughter thing isn't great, but this is another example of a repressed queer person

---

1 See '"Queer" history: A history of Queer' by Mollie Clarke, The National Archives: https://blog.nationalarchives.gov.uk/queer-history-a-history-of-queer/

attempting to navigate life as a repressed queer parent in a repressed heteronormative world. It's all so repressed!

So queer people can and will continue to forge families through various means. We can have children as a result of opposite-sex relationships. We can co-parent. In later years, we will adopt and foster. Technology will become a vital part of queer family building. But most importantly, we are good parents. Research consistently shows that queer parents are just as capable as heterosexual parents and that our children are just as healthy, both physically and mentally.

Queer parents are just as competent caregivers as non-queer parents. We're not running around in rainbow colours talking about smashing the gender binary while changing our children's nappies. I mean, some of us are, but mostly we're just trying to raise our children as best we can in a world that often makes things difficult.

As for me, I can recite almost every single episode of *Peppa Pig*. I've extracted snot from my son's nose using my mouth, and I've had his shit in my hair, behind my ear and weirdly in my belly button (though that might have been my own). I am just as much a parent as any other person; me being queer has absolutely nothing to do with my parenting (for context, my son *does* have an incredible sense of humour and looks like my shrunken twin).

I had always wanted children but had conditioned myself to believe that I couldn't. I had also been brainwashed into believing that bringing a child into this world would be selfish and dangerous for the child. This was drilled into me so much that it is still something that I struggle with today. I worry that my son will resent me for his existence or wish that he had a 'normal' family. There's a sense of guilt that will probably never leave me fully, but through the research for this book I have found that I am not alone, and never have been. Queer parents have been raising children and redefining the parameters of family forever. So let's go look at some more examples, shall we?

LESBIANS BEING LESBIANS

Seeing as I am a lesbian (surprise!), and I know lesbian history reasonably well, it seems appropriate to start with that – and where better than San Francisco? It was in San Francisco, during the mid-1950s, that Rosalie 'Rose' Bamberger announced that she would form her very own private lesbian social club. She wanted a place to discuss lesbian politics, the social structure of the patriarchy, and crazy ex-girlfriends (who were also probably in the lesbian social club, because you know… we love to shit where we eat).

The club's first meeting was held in 1955 at Rose's house and included the likes of Rose's girlfriend Rosemary Sliepen, Del Martin and her girlfriend Phyllis Lyon, along with some other lesbian couples.

As years passed, the group eventually morphed into the Daughters of Bilitis, a political group that went on to produce one of the first lesbian magazines in the USA, *The Ladder*. If you want to know more about the Daughters of Bilitis, why not buy my first book, *A Short History of Queer Women*, from Gay's the Word or Amazon, depending on your ethics!

As well as the patriarchy, fingering and loose underwear, the group discussed motherhood. This was Del Martin's idea because by then she was divorced (from a man) and had one daughter (from the same man). This man also had primary custody.

Del wanted the struggles of lesbian motherhood to be widely discussed. She wrote articles on lesbians raising children from former heterosexual relationships and published them in *The Ladder*. She purposefully sought essays and papers on women raising children with other women. Finally, along with her pal Pat Norman, she formed the Lesbian Mothers Union (LMU).

Shoutout to Pat

In 1977, Pat Norman and three of her children were featured in *In the Best Interest of Children*, a documentary that focused on eight lesbian mothers, their children and the custody battles they went through. The documentary was groundbreaking in that it not only interviewed and highlighted the lesbian mothers involved but also, for the first time, featured the opinions and (often hilarious) thoughts of their children.

For instance, when asked how being a lesbian had changed their mother, one child replied, 'She's a lot happier...'

Yeah, I bet she is, we're all happier when we become lesbians, just ask my girlfriend. (I hope her ex-husband doesn't read this... or do I?)

Another kid quipped, 'I know about more things than other kids.'

Yeah, I bet they did. Like how pocket chains are genuinely practical and not just stylish.

It was a film made by lesbians for lesbians but also for the rest of the world to see that lesbian mothers were good people and not incapable of looking after their kids. Most importantly, it sympathised with lesbians – it made audiences feel sad for us! It told people how lesbians were routinely forced to undergo psychological testing to prove that they weren't a danger to their children and how they had to constantly deal with homophobic judges and misogynistic courts. It made lesbians look 'normal' – to an extent. I mean, between you and me, we're all batshit. But don't tell the judge!

Pat Norman was especially important to the documentary. Not only had she spent a long time fighting for the custody of her *own* children, but as a Black lesbian, her voice was vital. This was because back then (and often now) lesbian motherhood was/is mostly discussed within a white, middle-class context, which is annoying because, believe it or not, lesbians and queer people who are not white or middle class also have children.

It was around this time that Pat was employed as the first openly lesbian San Francisco Health Department employee. She then created the position of Coordinator of Lesbian/Gay Health Services and became heavily involved in the community's response to the AIDS epidemic during the 1980s. Meanwhile, I'm sitting here in my underwear, eating biscuits and worrying about finishing a book that I willingly chose to write.

Pat identified as a lesbian, and she had a long-term partner. She had six children, as well as grandchildren and great-grandchildren. She forged a family unit and fought for their rights every day. She also did a million other things for her family and for the community that led to her being recognised and portrayed by Whoopi Goldberg in the television series *When We Rise* (2017).

But let's get back to the Lesbian Mothers Union. The LMU highlighted the various legal issues that lesbian mothers were facing at the time. The main issue, as always, was the C-word. *Custody* (gotcha!).

During the 1970s, queer mothers all over the United States were having their children taken away from them on the sole basis that they were queer. So, the LMU would provide financial and legal aid to mothers who needed to pay for lawyers, court fees and dildos because a lesbian *really* needs to get off during a custody battle.

To raise funds, they held Lesbian Mothers' Day Auctions – selling second-hand copies of Radclyffe Hall's *The Well of Loneliness* and thoroughly polished strap-ons. They would research medical histories in the hope that it would demonstrate that lesbian mothers were just the same as straight mothers only with shorter nails and a better sense of humour. They also introduced lesbian mothers to other lesbian mothers so that they could take over the world with their blended lesbian families and abundance of plaid shirts.

But, given the world we live in, a lesbian group founded by a butch lesbian (hi, Del) and a Black lesbian (shoutout to Pat) was never going to last and, like all good causes, they eventually disbanded. But don't fret, because other groups were inspired by them…

See you in court

One such group was the Lesbian Mothers National Defense Fund, which was founded in 1974 to help lesbian mothers embroiled in nasty custody disputes. The thing that made this group a little different was that they also set out to educate lesbians and queers about having children and, in many ways, introduced the notion that it was an option.

They brought lesbian parents together with other lesbians who wanted to know how to have kids. They printed pamphlets on donor insemination and legal rights. To be honest, I could have done with the LMNDF, because when I realised that I might want to have a child, I had no idea where to start, what to do, or who to talk to.

The LMNDF held fundraisers to help with legal fees and even had a newsletter named *Mom's Apple Pie*, which is exactly what I'd expect a lesbian motherhood newsletter to be called, that or 'Lez Be Moms' – feel free to DM me with alternatives!

One famous LMNDF case involved lesbian couple Sandy Schuster and Madeleine Isaacson, who were sued by their husbands. Now, I know husbands aren't always bad, and that there are some nice husbands out there, but those husbands are not in this book, at least not in this chapter.

Sandy and Madeleine first met at church, which for some reason makes this story even gayer. Instead of learning about God (is that what happens in church?) the pair fell in love and left their husbands.

The husbands were upset, which is understandable, especially when someone leaves you for someone else, but that's why we have ice cream, that's why people write godawful poetry and sleep with inappropriate people and immediately regret it. Maybe that's just me speaking, but my point is to not do anything too vindictive… like humiliate or sue your ex-wife, the mother of your children.

When they got to court, Sandy and Madeleine were made to feel like terrible mothers who were a danger to their kids for being gay and in love. In a shocking twist, they were each eventually granted custody of their *own* children but were specifically told that they must not move their families into one house. This judge obviously hadn't heard of the lesbian urge to merge.

So, what did Sandy Schuster and Madeleine Isaacson do? They did what any other ingenious lesbians would do: they found two separate apartments across the hall from one another and moved in with their families. Like if *Friends* ditched the heteros and focused on Carol and Susan instead. OMG, sign me up!

The husbands didn't like this. Of course they didn't, because nothing irritates a straight man more than a clever woman. So what did they do? They sued their wives *again*. This then turned into another lengthy court battle that included twenty-one witnesses, eleven psychiatrists and psychologists, three French hens...

In the end, the court eventually decided that 'almost all of the testimony of all the people who actually saw, examined, or talked to the children was that the children are healthy, happy, normal, loving children' – oh, and that they could remain with their mothers. How about that for a waste of time, money and emotional energy?

Sadly, other parents were not as 'lucky' – with the courtroom suddenly becoming a character in its own right, not because queers love the drama (which we do) but because a Christian patriarchal world just hates to be threatened.

Take Marilyn Koop, a woman who had two of her three children taken away from her. The reason? The judge just couldn't understand why her children would want to stay with a lesbian rather than with their straight father. The kids were eventually placed in a detention centre because they actively refused to stay with their father... YES, THEY REFUSED. But a refusal from the childrens' mouths was seemingly not enough and the judge was all like, 'Why do you want to live with your mother and her girlfriend in such "abnormal" and "highly detrimental" living arrangements?'

Now, when the children are choosing to stay in a detention centre over living with their father... this to me suggests that there is a problem with the father. But then what I do know? I'm just a batshit lesbian.

Speaking of batshit lesbians, courts often used anything they could to make mothers appear 'unfit', especially the more feminist-leaning mothers. In one case, a woman who had feminist literature in her home was accused of influencing her daughter by creating an 'exotic atmosphere in which intellectual opinions expressing themselves as an eagerness for total feminine freedom, sexual and otherwise, will have a marked influence' – she sounds like my mother and she's the straightest person in the world. No offence, Mum. The court then went on to say that the woman's daughters would 'be exposed to propaganda about sexual morality which could expose them to quite extraordinary risks in adolescence' – well, I'm pretty sure that the risks in adolescence are coming from horny boys and a culture of toxic masculinity, and definitely *not* female relationships. But then again, what do I know? I grew up watching Britney Spears be both virgin pin-up and a legal prisoner, so clearly the whole idea of role models and narratives is all just a bit... off.

It then took until 1974 for a New Jersey court judge to decide that a person's sexuality (in this case a gay man) was no reason to deny child visitation. It was a groundbreaking decision: one of the first pronouncements that a person's sexuality was deemed unimportant when it came to parenting their children.

It actually took two more years for the United States to stop judges from making custody rulings based on a person's sexual orientation, but even after that, a judge's bias still influenced their decision-making. You see, being a queer parent, or even just a queer person, is mostly about heterosexuals telling you what they can and cannot abide. #notallheterosexuals.

As previously mentioned, many lesbians and queer people had children in the context of their heterosexual marriages. Many had rings on their fingers and children before even realising they were queer. But, by then, it was often too late for them to leave. Being married meant financial security, and a home, especially for women. Leaving your husband usually meant losing your kids.

You only need to read this letter to the lesbian magazine *Sappho* in 1978 to see what I mean.

Have any of you out lesbians thought how lucky you are? You would call me bisexual because I live with my husband. I live with him because I have two children and they love him. What right do I have to take them away from him? I don't leave because I could not live without my children. I live an empty, lonely life and deserve an Oscar for my acting ability and the length of it.[2]

I love how queer people habitually declare that they deserve awards, something as true in 1978 as today. I deserve a Pulitzer for writing this book! But the letter writer was right, and she wasn't the only one.

A few years earlier (1967), the current-affairs television series *Man Alive* explored homosexuality in the United Kingdom in a two-part report called 'Consenting Adults'. The second episode, 'The Women', featured various lesbians trying to navigate their way through life. The documentary was surprisingly sympathetic for the time and portrayed the women as individuals just trying to fit into a society that wouldn't accept them. Even Angela Huth's introduction was quite... nice?

There is no legal frown on their relationships. No parliamentary discussion about their behaviour. And yet for women who love women unqualified acceptance by our society still does not exist. We are heterosexuality geared, naturally propaganda for love, and sex,

---

2 Letter from J.H., Cheshire, to *Sappho* (1978).

for conformist lives all aimed at women with men. The idea of two women feeling about each other in the same way as a normal couple disturbs that happy concept. And so, lesbians receive the minority treatment – intolerance, suspicion, often disgust. The fact that they are legally free to live as they like makes little difference.

There were, of course, a few problematic parts. This was nearly sixty years ago, after all. At one point, we are introduced to two women who are clearly very happy and in love. Ange, God bless her, then asks every straight person's favourite question: 'Is one of you the predominant figure like the man?'

For fuck's sake, Angela, you had one job!

At the end of the documentary, we meet a woman who is married to a man. She identifies as a lesbian and is very content with that because it's great being a lesbian, isn't it?… Isn't it!

Angela: Have you ever actually faced having to make this decision, between a woman and staying with your husband?

Woman: Yes.

Angela: What did you decide?

Woman: I decided to go. I was perfectly prepared to do so. In fact, I was once looking for a flat. I was going to take my younger son with me because, I think, when one is fourteen, and he has been through a tough time, of course, one needs one's mother still. But as it always happens, or it always seems to happen to me, at any rate… you know, they can't take it, the other women. The possessiveness is so tremendous that the thing breaks up, because you are not acceptable as a married woman. You have got a family, you belong to somebody else. Even if you deny belonging to your husband, you cannot deny that you belong to your children. Indeed, you don't want to deny that you belong to your children. You visualise the kind of existence where you can live your life with your chosen partner and yet still participate in the lives that your children lead, even though they may get married, you may want to see the grandchildren. This is something that your partner cannot accept.

Angela: Do the neighbours know about you here?

Woman: I don't know, and I don't care. My neighbours must think me an odd bird, anyway. Because I'm different, I know. But I don't care what they think. The only reason why I would care was in case it should injure my husband or the children… It hurts me when they laugh and when they sneer.

Angela: Do they do that in front of you?

Woman: Oh, yes, indeed they do, this is something that people cannot understand. They think that being a

homosexual is something odd. They think it is filthy, perhaps, even disgusting, which it isn't of course. There
is nothing at all extraordinary in being a homosexual,
any more than there is in being heterosexual. It's the
sneering that I can't get. And 'digs', as they say. And
the laughing. The funny speculation, I wonder what
they do in bed with each other. You know?

The interview ends with the woman explaining
how after each relationship ends, she has the same
thoughts over and over again.

So, suddenly, I found myself again with empty hands.
Wondering why in hell I was ever born. And there isn't
anything I can do. I can only look forward to another
twenty years of life, perhaps twenty-five if I'm unlucky
enough to live as long as that. Never finding what
I want… and living with a man who has no hope of
ever being able to establish the kind of relationship
that he wants with me. Nothing, in fact, nothing but
the wilderness without love.

I can't really follow that up with anything witty, so
there it is.

Time for a little positivity… (to an extent)

Back in the USA, in the late 1970s, San Francisco
lawyers Donna Hitchens (the first openly gay

elected female judge in the United States) and Roberta Achtenberg formed the Lesbian Rights Project. Lesbians *love* a project.

The project later became the National Center for Lesbian Rights (NCLR), confirming what we always knew... lesbians go fucking nuts for acronyms. The NCLR went on to help many LGBTQIA+ families across the United States and became the largest national lesbian organisation ever by numbers. Not counting Cate Blanchett's lesbian following on Insta, of course.

Roberta Achtenberg was the first out official to be confirmed in her position by the United States Senate – as the assistant secretary for Housing and Urban Development. She got a lot of support from her colleagues, friends and the general public when she came out. She also got a lot of criticism from religious Republican politicians, which surprised absolutely nobody because religious Republican politicians love to ruin a gay party.

To infuriate the Republicans even more, Roberta entered into a relationship with Mary Morgan, a judge on the San Francisco Municipal Court. They were the ultimate lesbian power couple.

Roberta and Mary went on to have a child together and became one of the most visibly queer families in the United States. This family were unique at that point in that Roberta and Mary actively chose to have this child. It was not a child from a previous heterosexual relationship – it was a child they deliberately chose to have, together.

Michele Zavos and her partner Libby Leader did the same thing in the early 1980s. They were celebrating their thirtieth birthdays and, like most twenty-nine-year-olds, they had felt THE FEAR. The fear that they weren't doing anything with their lives. What was life anyway? Was anything meaningful anymore, did anything *really* matter? Who even wants a family? Is it unethical to even bring a child into this world? Sorry, that was *my* twenty-ninth-birthday fear, not Michele and Libby's. But Michele and Libby did want children. At least they thought they did.

Michele and Libby had never really discussed having children before, because, well, they were brought up in a country where that wasn't an option for them. They also didn't know any other lesbians who had purposefully had children together. I say purposefully because, as we have learnt, many queer people had families that pre-dated their sexual awakenings.

So, what did Michelle and Libby do? Here are some clues.

1 They were lesbians.
2 They wanted to discuss a very serious political issue.

They started a lesbian political group! The group met every Tuesday and discussed everything from assimilating to heteronormativity, adoption, gender, fertility centres, and all the light-hearted and fun topics you would expect from a lesbian political group in the 1980s. But one question came up time and time again. No, not what acronym they should use, but what the fuck were they going to do about sperm?

SPERM ME ON

The late 1970s showed a noticeable change in how lesbians and queer people were having their children. While many were still blending families from previous heterosexual relationships, others were now embarking on a new chapter, artificial insemination (AI; also known as intrauterine insemination).

We now recognise AI as shorthand for artificial intelligence – you know, like the kind that wrote this book. But here, let's talk about artificial insemination. AI is basically when sperm is injected into a person's womb in the hope they will get pregnant. It was first used for people who, for whatever reason, could not or did not want to engage in vaginal intercourse. These days it's often used by queer people (either alone or in relationships) and straight women who have had enough of straight men and their bullshit. I met a lot of these people on my IVF journey (hey, Sarah!).

Access to AI depends on where you live in the world. It's also really cheap! Joke: it's mad expensive. But we'll talk about that later; first let's talk about sperm, said no lesbian ever.

In 1978, the *London Evening News* took it upon themselves to inform their readers that British lesbians and queers were having children... with each other!

'But how?' the British public asked.

'Through artificial insemination,' the *London Evening News* responded.

'And what is artificial insemination?' the British public asked.

'We don't really know,' the *London Evening News* replied. 'But they are doing it!'

The paper explained that queer people (mainly those dastardly lesbians) were planning on raising children, all while challenging conventional family models and the idea that lesbianism and motherhood were mutually exclusive... It was indeed possible to do both. Yay! Women really *can* have it all!

As you can imagine, this spawned a few opinions. I say opinions, but what I really mean is mass homophobia. The story was then brought to Parliament because, of course, queer parenting and lesbian motherhood should only ever be talked about by straight, white, elderly men.

You see, back then, the British public was still struggling to understand homosexuality as a concept, never mind the fact that lesbians were now having children via some outlandish technology that nobody really understood. A baby? Without a man? Unheard of. Even the queers didn't get it. Sure, the lesbians were overjoyed – but they were still suspicious. Having children without a man was the dream, but could it really be possible?

On Tuesday nights in Notting Hill...

It was around this time that British lesbian Jackie Forster helped form the lesbian social group called, er, Sappho. The group met every Tuesday in Notting Hill, west London, to discuss things that lesbians had to deal with in the 1970s... like homosexuality being listed as a mental disorder, like being excluded from second-wave feminism, and like where to get the best enamel pins.

At that time, Jackie Forster was living with her partner, Babs Todd (a name that could only ever be given to a queer person), and Babs's two young children. Jackie began discussing her living situation openly in meetings and soon realised that she wasn't the only queer person who had happily 'inherited' children. She also realised that more and more queer people were becoming vocal about wanting children, not as a result of previous hetero relationships but together, as in together together. They wanted children with their partners and they wanted to make them *together*.

Then, during one Tuesday-night meeting, a mysterious Australian lesbian couple showed up. I don't know where I've got 'mysterious' from, but it adds intrigue, right? The conversation once again turned to children, and the mysterious Australian lesbian couple suggested a ground-breaking option.

'Why don't you try artificial insemination by donor?' Aussie 1 said.

'I've never heard of that,' said Jackie.

'Well, Britain, and I think Sweden, are the only two countries where there needs to be no consent by a husband. So single women, especially lesbian couples, can get it. But you know, you need a gynae-cologist,' Aussie 2 said.

'We've got one actually,' Aussie 1 said.

'Well, do you suppose they'd come to the next meeting and tell us about it?' Jackie said.

They came, they thawed, they conquered

Despite the lack of knowledge expressed by Jackie Forster, along with the rest of the United Kingdom (and the rest of the world), artificial insemination as a medical procedure had been around a lot longer than most people could comprehend.

As far back as 1866, you had Italian scientist Paolo Mantegazza freezing his sperm, unfreezing it four days later, then realising that it was still alive. Paolo's discovery eventually led to sperm storage, and sperm banks, an integral part of fertility treatments today. Nice one, Paolo; for once I'm grateful for the weird shit that men get up to in their man caves.

But even before Paolo, you had Lazaro Spallanzani, a young Italian priest/physiologist (classic combo) who figured out that there must be physical contact between an egg and sperm for an embryo to develop. People already knew that and accused him of just mansplaining conception, so he went even further with his newfound 'discovery' and inseminated a dog (with dog sperm, to be clear), which resulted in the birth of three puppies. Does it make me bad for feeling more emotionally drawn to the puppy story than a successful insemination story about lesbians? I think it just makes me gayer.

Not long after, Scottish anatomist and surgeon (a more understandable combination of jobs) Dr John Hunter claimed that he had successfully inseminated a woman using her husband's sperm. What's strange here is that nobody seemed to want to know any more details and just took his word for it. Ah, to be a white man with wispy grey hair.

It took another hundred years for artificial insemination to be mentioned again, when a letter emerged in the North American journal *Medical World* stating that donor insemination had been performed in Philadelphia, USA. The people involved were a straight Quaker married couple who couldn't have kids because the wife was fifteen years older than the husband. It's always our fault!

The Quaker couple went to a doctor who subjected the wife to hundreds of invasive and unnecessary examinations that uncovered absolutely nothing. As a last resort, the husband was examined. Guess what? Sterile.

The doctor couldn't believe it, so he brought the case to the attention of his medical students. The class decided that *they* would be the ones to help impregnate the woman, suggesting that they collect sperm from the hottest person in the class and then inseminate the woman with attractive and sexy sperm.

Now at this point, you'd expect the doctor to say:

'That is a silly idea and ethically wrong. It's also probably illegal.'

But instead, he said:

'Great idea! And let's do it without telling her, haha!'

The doctor then collected the sperm from the 'hottest' student in the class, told the woman he was conducting a routine examination, and then inseminated sperm into her without her knowledge or permission. Nobody bothered to inform the husband either.

A few months later, the woman was pregnant. The couple were suspicious, so they returned to the doctor and asked him if he had done anything unruly while examining her. The doctor ignored her and asked to see the husband in another room. He then explained that he had instructed the hottest student in his class to spunk into a cup which he had then inseminated into the wife.

Now again, at this point, you'd expect the husband to say:

'That is very illegal and morally wrong. I'm going to contact the authorities and have your medical licence revoked.'

But instead, he said:

'That's great! I'm thrilled! And let's never tell my wife, haha!'

Once again we see that the world has so little regard for women and their bodies. But at least we can understand how artificial insemination started, how it works and how it has now become a crucial element in a queer person's parenting journey. Thanks to that morally bankrupt doctor who would probably be livid that gays are now benefiting from all this!

But for me, I wasn't really bothered about sperm banks, no matter what an important landmark they were. I knew I needed sperm, but I didn't care much about where it came from. As a lesbian, believe it or not, I rarely think about sperm. It also freaks me out slightly, but that, reader, is a story for my therapist.

Weirdly, as soon as word got out that we were trying to have a baby, the majority of cis men in my life started offering up their sperm. Like, just casually, in conversation, like they thought I was running a sperm drive or something. When I talked to other couples trying for a baby, they had the same experience, as if every man they knew believed that their sperm was some kind of miracle juice just waiting to be shared.

But to my complete surprise (and horror), choosing sperm became a highlight of the whole parenting journey and soon became central to every single conversation. How do we even get it? Where do we find it? And what about the donor? Is he going to appear at Christmas with a present saying, 'Love from Dad'? The answer was no, he wouldn't, because in the UK, and with the service we used (the European Sperm Bank), the donor essentially signs away all rights to any child produced from their sperm, so they're not legally the father. But, of course, as with everything in the queer parenting world, every country has different laws and legal rights, depending on how homophobic it is.

Back to the shopping. It was like Amazon but more expensive and with longer delivery times. I knew one couple who had to wait a further three months for their sperm delivery because it had got stuck at customs. Brexit, apparently!

Many people also like to pretend that they don't care what their child looks like, as long as they are happy and healthy. They are lying, because when you start choosing sperm there is so much choice that it makes it impossible *not* to care.

Most sperm banks provide baby pictures of the donor so you can try to imagine what they might look like now and how those genes could mix with your own. My son is biologically related to me, which, unfortunately for him, meant he was going to inherit some of my traits. So, who did I choose? A baby with a small nose, large eyes and great teeth.

You can also see how many babies a donor has produced, in other words, how many times their seed worked (I've been so desperate to write the word 'seed'). But don't worry, they are shelved after a specific number of successful inseminations, so it's unlikely that your child will run into their brother or sister on the next street, unless, you know... you're in Stoke Newington.

As you might guess, many queer people worry that the sperm donor will somehow have legal rights to their child. So I want to say this again. They don't. They aren't the baby's father, or a legal guardian, they are nothing but a bunch of cells. In the UK, the donor has no legal rights whatsoever, but the child *does* have a legal right to the details of their donor after turning eighteen and can contact them if they so wish. Does this bother me? I guess I should say no. I mean, I don't want to frighten prospective parents, but let's be honest, sharing my son with my ex-wife is hard enough, never mind some random man too.

Plus, it doesn't help that to this day, people still refer to my son's donor as the father. A father and a donor are not the same thing, unless you are a straight couple and the donor is the father, because then they are... but you know what I mean.

A father is a person who is involved in a child's upbringing. I understand that, without the donor, I wouldn't have my son, but a father is someone who is present, who watches them grow up, who loses sleep, goes without food, gets pissed on, shat on, thrown up on. The donor does not get to share those joys.

Ethical schmethical

As artificial insemination became more widespread, so did the question of ethics. Was it morally acceptable to interfere with the reproduction process? Was it OK to inseminate women without their permission or knowledge? Were these new developments in technology dangerous to women? Is the prospective child's health at risk with these methods? Questions you would expect to hear, right? No, the questions weren't centred around women's or children's safety but rather around whether or not these women could be seen to have committed adultery. Now I've heard everything.

And where did these questions come from? Why, the Vatican! The Roman Catholic Church was concerned that artificial insemination meant that women were technically cheating on their partners by housing someone else's sperm. They also said that it 'promoted the vice of masturbation' because sperm makes people SO HORNY. The conversation went back and forth before they realised they had other things to worry about.

Then, in the United States, a court of law claimed that a child conceived through donor insemination was illegitimate because the sperm donor was not married to the child's mother. The donor was considered the legal father and the only way to make the child 'legitimate' was for the donor to sign away the rights to the child and for the husband to officially adopt the child. Of course, this could never happen because a) no one had access to donor records, so the donor could not be contacted, and b) many husbands were already feeling emasculated because they couldn't get their wives pregnant to begin with, so they didn't want the added stigma of officially admitting the child wasn't theirs. So they would occasionally leave their wife and child in lieu of raising the child as their own.

Anyway – all this fragile masculinity is giving me wrinkles. Let's go back to Tuesday nights in Notting Hill.

Now that Jackie Forster had been made aware of artificial insemination, she decided to organise further meetings so that lesbians and queer people could learn more about it and how to use it. She then invited the mysterious gynaecologist recommended by the mysterious Australian lesbian couple to share a story about another lesbian couple who had come to him requesting artificial insemination. He contacted the chairman of the British Medical Association's

Ethical Committee about this request. The chairman was completely bewildered by the question because not once had he, or anybody else, ever thought to include queer people in their fertility narrative.

The chairman confirmed that, while there were no legal barriers, it was not respectable… in other words, no, queer people should not exercise the same rights as heterosexual people.

The gynaecologist went back to the group and explained that he didn't give a shit nor care about how it was morally wrong… at least that's what he said in my head. Are you ready for a story? Because this one is wild.

Dr. Strangelove, a brilliant ally

Dr David M. Sopher (did anyone else first read this as 'Sappho'?) was a respected gynaecologist based in Belgravia, central London. He helped many lesbians/queers have children through the use of artificial insemination.

Picture the scene. Great Britain during the early 1970s and Jackie Forster and Dr Sopher were running around Belgravia like Batman and Robin, only more masculine…

It usually went like this: Jackie would refer couples to Dr Sopher, who would then discreetly help them from his practice. In the beginning, Dr Sopher would meet with the couples and carry out full examinations on the person who would be getting pregnant. These examinations were legit, no molestation, no insemination without permission, everybody knew what was going on, just completely above-board examinations. It really is a shame that I have to say that, isn't it?

Dr Sopher would then provide the couples with donor sperm (which had been tested and given the all-clear) and then inseminate the patient using a private room in his clinic. He soon realised that getting your hands on sperm was rather difficult and that the couples could probably do the insemination part themselves. So, to help move things along and to help more people, he encouraged them to find their own sperm (which he would still test) and then to inseminate themselves (which he would show them how to do).

What does a lesbian bring on a first date? A turkey baster!

You might think the turkey baster joke is, well… just a joke, but it's actually one of the oldest home-insemination methods. You see, women may be imaginative when it comes to getting pregnant but they are also very practical, so when I say turkey baster, I don't specifically mean a real turkey baster (not always anyway) but something of that ilk.

TURKEY BASTER METHOD

How to use a turkey baster to get pregnant (imagined by someone who has never used one)

1   Get sperm (with consent).
2   Put sperm into turkey baster (wear gloves and do *not* let that sperm touch you).
3   Spread legs (you might need the help of someone else?).
4   Get horny (see above).
5   Transfer sperm into the vagina (without laughing).
6   Lie down for half an hour (naptime).
7   Pregnant!

Jackie liked that lesbians and queers could inseminate themselves at home, so she also encouraged others to do it. She then got a load of lesbians together and tasked them with getting more sperm. They called themselves the Fairy Godmothers (God I love lesbians).

The Fairy Godmothers began storing sperm wherever they could, from home freezers to office fridges to bathtubs filled with ice. Who knows what else they did, but lesbians are smart, so you can only imagine some of the other ingenious things they came up with to store that shit.

Lesbians are smart, but they are fucking terrible at keeping secrets. Jackie regularly shared stories about Dr Sopher, the Fairy Godmothers and artificial insemination in the magazine *Sappho*. She also discussed it openly during the Tuesday evening meetings. Any guesses as to what happened next?

Joanna Patnya was an undercover reporter for the *London Evening News*. She'd heard rumblings about lesbians churning out babies without men so decided to attend a Tuesday night meeting undercover. Her undercover name... Joanna Allison.

Look, I'm not an undercover journalist, nor am I a secret agent, but I've watched enough BBC dramas to know that when you go undercover, you change your first name too, Jo!

As you'd expect, Joanna immediately made a beeline for Jackie. Joanna lied to Jackie about having a best friend who she was in love with, which then turned into a happy relationship – the classic lesbian 'how did you guys get together?' story. She then explained that they wanted children but didn't know how to go about that... could you help, Jackie? Do you know anyone? Jackie being Jackie was happy to help a dyke in need. She then told Joanna all about Dr Sopher, his practice, the Fairy Godmothers, the sperm, everything.

Joanna booked an appointment with Dr Sopher and told him the same story. He asked her some questions about relationships and periods, then told her that the fee was £12 per insemination (a lot less than the £7,000 that I paid in 2021). He also told her that Harley Street doctors were charging the straights £150 a pop and that he 'believed he was providing a worthwhile service on the grounds... that the alternative of indulging in a casual heterosexual relationship would be abhorrent'.

Honestly, the more I read about Dr Sopher, the more I love him and the more I want him to inseminate me. Unfortunately, for every Dr Sopher, you have a thousand wrong 'uns, like this knob, Cecil Jacobson.

Mr Fertility Fraud

Around the same time, American quack doctor Cecil Jacobson was running a fertility clinic in the southern US state of Virginia. Cecil would inject his patients with hCG (a hormone normally released during pregnancy) before and after conception.

This was met with a lot of success, or at least that's what he led his patients to believe.

In fact, after inseminating his clients, he would then perform an ultrasound that supposedly showed a foetus. The women all reported bodily changes and truly believed that they were pregnant. They weren't. In reality, the changes were just bodily reactions to the hCG and Cecil's 'ultrasounds' showed either other organs or faecal matter.

Cecil was sued by several patients and eventually arrested. It was then revealed that Cecil had been using his *own* sperm to inseminate the women. ARGH! Overall, he was suspected of 'fathering' over seventy-five children including a patient who had provided the sperm of her husband. His medical licence was revoked, and he was sentenced to five years in prison because that's considered fair in a misogynist world.

During the trial, Jacobson acknowledged that he had used his own sperm for artificial insemination when other, anonymous donors were not available. When asked why, he reasoned that his own fresh sperm was better than any frozen sperm from a sperm bank. I mean, of course he fucking did.

But enough of him. Back to the lovely Dr Sopher, for whom things were starting to unravel.

Joanna Allison announced she had been Joanna Patnya all along and the story was dropped on an unsuspecting, heterosexual, general public. As expected, it caused a humungous media sensation and, as mentioned earlier, a conversation in Parliament.

Conservative MP Dame Jill Knight said, 'I am not concerned with the lifestyle of the lesbians, nor would I condemn them. But it is very worrying from the point of view of the children that this should be permitted.'

Thus, showing that she *was* concerned with the lifestyle of lesbians and that she *would* condemn them.

Another Tory ******* shadow minister, Sir Rhodes Boyson, said, 'To bring children into this world without a natural father is evil and selfish. This evil must stop for the sake of the potential children and society, which both have enough problems without the extension of this horrific practice.'

This from a man who loved corporal punishment so much that his nickname was the 'Minister for Flogging' – this from a man who said, 'AIDS is the part of the fruits of the permissive society. The regular one-man, one-woman marriage would not put us at risk in this way. If we could wipe out homosexual practices, then AIDS would die out.'

This from a guy who called *us* evil.

But it wasn't just straight people in Parliament giving us their unwanted opinions, other straight people felt the need to express their unwanted opinions too.

A man called Dr Dilcas Short said, 'Every child has as great a need for a father as a mother to allow for normal growth, and to gain emotional balance. What chance would a child have in a lesbian household, to become balanced and happy?'

A man still holding a grudge at being named Dilcas.

Fleet Street journo Jean Rook also declared that lesbians were not fit mothers (get a new insult, Jean!) and described a lesbian relationship as 'more neurotic, passionate, jealous and highly-sexed than a standard marriage'.

What's your point, Jean!

As a result, Dr Sopher went into hiding and many couples who had consulted with him were fearful for their lives and their children's lives. But as you may know, you mess with a queer person, you mess with us all, and Joanna Patyna's London flat was soon spray-painted with the words 'Lesbian Mums are OK!' Look, I said lesbians were smart, I didn't say that they had imagination...

But it wasn't all bad: the article meant that lesbians and queer people near and far were now aware of artificial insemination and what that could mean for their futures. Jackie Forster's Tuesday night group was inundated with curious queers enquiring about where they could get sperm and how they could put it inside them without having to touch a penis.

The *London Evening News* became obsessed with lesbians and queer relationships and quickly published another piece about a woman named 'Helen' and her two lovers. No, it wasn't a porno.

Helen was living in London with her lover Julie and Julie's other lover Alison. See! People were cool and fluid long before Gen Z! Helen had conceived her son through artificial insemination and the decision was made to have all three women look after him.

When their child was born, there were some 'misunderstandings' or as I like to call it, knobhead behaviour. For instance, Helen was put into a special ward because she was an 'unmarried mother' – unmarried she may have been, but she still had two girlfriends, oi, oi. Then when it came to registering their son's birth, the registrar was, in Julie's words, 'pretty snooty' – change the word 'pretty' to 'giant' and 'snooty' to 'prick' and you've got the doctor who asked me who my son's male role models would be two hours after he was born.

When asked what she would do when Michael asked about his father, Helen said, 'We'll say, "No, darling, you haven't got a Daddy but you have Julie and Alison instead, and they love you very much."'

And there you go. It's that fucking simple.

Speaking of the babies. In 1974, Babs Todd beautifully described meeting the Sappho group's first artificially inseminated baby, writing, 'I'm very grateful that I saw him on the day he was born. I don't think I have ever been so profoundly moved. It is not as if the miracle of birth is a new thing to me. I have two children of my own… When I came home, it struck me how I'd never been able to swallow the dogma of the Virgin Birth and how I'd never said, when reciting the Creed, the "born of the Virgin Mary" bit. And here he was – is – a Virgin Birth made possible by science. And I was allowed to hold him in my arms, and felt very proud and very humble.'

Forty-plus years later I had the same experience holding my own little baby boy, made possible by science, feeling proud and eternally grateful to those that came before me.

HOW DO YOU LIKE
YOUR EGGS?

On 25 July 1978 Louise Joy Brown became the first person to be born after being conceived outside of the human body, through in vitro fertilisation (IVF). We've all heard of IVF but what exactly is it? Well, it's basically the scientific equivalent of online dating but for eggs and sperm. You throw both of them together (in a dish), hope they get along, and then, if you're lucky, you might get laid – or in this case produce a baby. Look, I'm not a scientist – I'm just a semi-competent writer who compares everything to love and sex because, honestly, it's the only analogy I can muster.

The British scientists Robert Edwards, Patrick Steptoe (and son?) and Jean Purdy were all responsible for this unbelievable accomplishment. Despite being the world's first embryologist and an essential member of the team, Jean's contributions have been forgotten, mainly due to her early death but also because she was, well, a woman. Despite this, Louise's birth was a great thing for many reasons.

1 It was an incredible achievement for science!
2 It helped people become parents!
3 Louise was British and even better... northern, Oldham at that!

The media went crazy for Louise's birth with people all over the world awaiting her arrival. *Time* magazine called it 'the most awaited birth in perhaps 2,000 years' – which was ironic because the religious groups were really uncomfortable with science 'playing God' and instead chose to believe that it was a muscular grandad in the sky who created the universe.

But it wasn't just religious groups; scientists were also a bit freaked out, with British geneticist Robert J. Berry saying, 'Western society is built around the family; once you divorce sex from procreation, what happens to the family?'

Well, it becomes a gay family, Robert! Cheers! For queer people, Louise's birth opened new means of parenting. Sure, lesbians were already adopting 'do it yourself' methods at home, but it wasn't really safe, nor was it always practical. And what about the rest of the community, where did they fit in?

When I first realised that I wanted children, I assumed that it would be by IVF even if I didn't really know what IVF was. I knew that it probably involved a hospital, some needles, and maybe some witchcraft, but the most important thing for me was that it meant a sperm-free existence.

I soon discovered that IVF was much more than a couple of needles and a hospital visit. Sadly, there was no witchcraft either, which, as a closet lesbian who'd watched *The Craft* on repeat, was a huge letdown. I was honestly just hoping for a dramatic spell or, at the very least, some interaction with a goth.

It was actually a lot more complicated than I had imagined. I was also forgetting something rather important: who would carry the baby to term? It certainly wasn't going to be me, was it?

I'd never had that *burning* maternal urge to be pregnant. The thought of carrying a baby seemed rather terrifying. I just couldn't picture myself pregnant – my brain and a pregnant body were basically on different planets. I also didn't think that I was mentally strong enough for it.

I remember having a real fear of pregnancy and childbirth when I was young. Sure, childbirth is scary, it's painful. It's the ripping your vagina in half, the rivers of bodily fluids, the fact that you might shit yourself – all while squeezing an actual human out of a hole that just shouldn't deliver anything that big. But even that bit I reckoned I could get through; it was the growing-a-person-inside-of-me part that I couldn't wrap my head around.

Pregnancy was the thing that messed with me. It wasn't just the obvious: the weight gain, the nausea, the feeling knackered all the time. It was a lot deeper than that. I didn't like the idea that I was going to become a version of myself that I didn't quite understand or even recognise. I am a cis woman, assigned female at birth, and very happy and lucky enough to feel comfortable with that. I love being a 'woman', whatever that may mean for me. But a pregnant woman was something I just couldn't get on board with.

For as long as I can remember, I haven't really *liked* my body. I would say that I have what would be described in the Western world as a 'womanly figure' – I have curves, wide hips, large(ish) boobs. It's a body that doesn't quite fit my chosen aesthetic. It doesn't match up with what I have going on in my head. Being pregnant, I assumed, would accentuate those features: my boobs would get bigger, my hips would get wider…

I questioned how this physical transformation would affect my identity and sense of self. Like, if I started to feel 'womanly', would I lose the part of me that had always felt more neutral? I had spent a good portion of my life battling gender stereotypes, trying to figure out how to exist in a world that wasn't particularly open to that, yet pregnancy felt like it would undo all that work.

Confusingly, I still wanted to have a child. I wanted one biologically and I don't think there is any shame in that, even if it is a bit *Game of Thrones*. I wanted to continue the family line. I don't have any brothers or sisters, and my mum's adopted, so the thought of my genetic line just… ending? I mean, someone has to continue the tradition of poor decisions and attachment issues, right?

So, as this is starting to sound dangerously Carrie Bradshaw, let's wrap up with some *real* and inspired wisdom from the feminist icon herself: 'Are we simply romantically challenged, or are we just… sluts?' – oh, wait, no, not that one. Here's the one *I* just came up with: 'I couldn't help but wonder… is pregnancy really the only route to motherhood?'

Enter reciprocal IVF, the heavenly chorus, spotlight, etc.

Reciprocal IVF (partner-assisted reproduction, or shared motherhood) is a fertility treatment for same-sex female couples to take part in the biological and gestational parts of pregnancy (one person's bun in another person's oven).

For me, reciprocal IVF was the universe saying, 'Hey, *bitch*, you can have your cake and eat it too.' Which, to be fair, was true, but I was also genuinely grateful for the whole thing. Science has no business being this clever.

I first stumbled across the concept of reciprocal IVF in my late twenties, and I didn't totally get it at the time (and to be honest, having done it, I still don't totally get it). I just remember reading about a lesbian couple who had a baby, and both of them were involved. BOTH OF THEM. It felt almost too perfect – where was the inevitable plot twist? Did we have to touch a penis? Was blowing someone in the small print?

What I liked was that this same-sex couple had made a baby together, out of love, no less. And while, let's be real, a baby being made out of love wasn't my top priority (I mean, I wasn't born out of love, I'm the product of a one-night stand), the idea that we, as a queer couple, could choose to have a baby together? Mind-blowing. It felt like we were finally getting close to the standard hetero baby-making ritual. You know, the one where the groupie sleeps with the guy in the band and everyone congratulates them for having a baby. Maybe that was just my conception story...

Also, don't get me wrong, I'm not saying that that is the only way to have a child, or even the 'correct' way, because what does 'correct' mean anyway? There is no 'correct' way. But for me, the idea that there was a possibility to have a child who was biologically related to me, and that my ex-wife and I could actually do this together – create something together – well, that was pretty special.

When I met my ex-wife, I had just come out of a long-term relationship. So, like every other lesbian, I thought, what would be the healthiest thing to do right now? Jump straight into another relationship, have a child and get married, obviously. As you can probably guess, things didn't work out, hence the 'ex' part of 'ex-wife' – but we did create the most perfect little boy to ever exist, so we did get something right.

Like I said, the only thing I knew about reciprocal IVF was a random article that I had read years before. I had a vague sense that it would be expensive and complicated, much like a single cup of coffee in Brighton or literally going anywhere with your toddler. But really, I had no idea what I was getting into. The information out there was perplexingly sparse but, at the same time, very overwhelming, so we decided to visit our local GP.

As you would expect, our local GP was about as helpful as a lesbian at a hen night. They weren't homophobic or dismissive, they just didn't know what was going on. Why were there inflatable dicks everywhere? Why is prosecco the only drink available? Why must we play fifty-five different versions of Mr and Mrs? Why is everything so LOUD? So. Many. Questions.

We both also really fancied her, which isn't relevant to the story but just an observation on how thirsty lesbians can be, especially for women in positions of power.

Still, I was a little shocked. I mean, we were in Brighton, surely it was a queer fertility theme park with 'make a baby' clinics sandwiched between the vegan cafés and sex shops. But no, instead she called some people higher up to enquire about funding. They replied by recommending that we start with a sperm sample to figure out why we were infertile. Didn't even need to come up with a joke for that one!

So, what did we do? We called the real experts of course, our exes. If there's one thing the queer community is really good at, it's remaining civil with ex-partners and sharing intel, especially when it's about surviving in a heteronormative world.

By doing this we learnt a lot, about artificial insemination, egg swapping, donor sperm, and all the different ways queer people could make a baby. We also realised that a clinic specialising in queer families was right on our doorstep. I say specialising… in the beginning they pretended that they did, but it was just some hardcore queer baiting designed to get the pink pound. Be careful of those.

We found out later that our clinic had some bad reviews. We then found out that my ex-wife's ex (honestly, find me a lesbian story without an ex) had also used this clinic and later complained, receiving compensation. We really should have seen that as a red flag, but this girl *did* get pregnant, and so did we (spoiler alert), and that's the eventual goal, right? That and the drama. BECAUSE I LIVE FOR IT.

What are the eggpsenses?

Really, the puns you can make with the word 'egg' are a gift to a writer who survives entirely on puns. Anyway, in 2007, the CEFER Institute in Barcelona, Spain, made headlines when they discovered a new way to make babies, because, you know, IVF just isn't complicated enough. This was reciprocal IVF, and, as mentioned, it was pretty much a game changer in terms of how queer people could have children.

Over in the UK, the Human Fertilisation and Embryology Authority (the fertility fun police) was set up in 1990 to oversee all things related to human embryos and fertility treatments. Their job was (and is) to license, monitor and inspect fertility clinics (and to make sure people weren't just winging it with a turkey baster and a prayer). I'm boring myself as I write this but it's important to mention because these are the people responsible for ensuring that patients get the best care, especially when you're spending thousands and thousands of pounds for a baby. And, of course, they also make sure you're legally protected. I mean, we are living in an actual apocalypse right now and the last thing you need is the government not recognising your family as legitimate.

So, if you're the same as me and prone to picturing dystopian nightmares where children from queer families are shipped off to 'normal' family camps, then welcome to my TED Talk. And yeah, you might be thinking, 'LOL, Kirsty, you're such a drama queen, relax.'

But if you're reading this book, you're probably queer, so instead of rolling your eyes, you're likely thinking, 'LOL, Kirsty, you're absolutely right' – because in Italy, non-biological parents are being erased from birth certificates, and in the United States, they're busy banning books and threatening teachers with jail time for daring to talk about anything other than 'traditional' families – they are also calling sports teams that win *American* leagues 'world' champions, and while that might be minor when compared to the other stuff, it's still unsettling.

But don't worry, I won't drag you through a full political meltdown (yet). Let's talk about the sexy part instead... the cost.

In 2021, a Stonewall and DIVA survey revealed that 36% of queer parents faced major barriers when starting their families. The biggest challenge? Money. Yes, financial access to IVF for queer people is a shitshow and, for some reason, people keep acting like funding for queer people is a new problem, one that isn't big enough to be acknowledged yet. But guess what, world, queer people want children, they always have. I can't believe I just wrote 'guess what, world' like a motivational speaker at a secondary-school assembly.

In the UK, depending on the method, costs can range from a few thousand pounds to tens of thousands. For most cis, straight people, fertility treatment is often a last resort because they've tried and not been able to procreate. Now, I'm not a scientist; nor am I a doctor. But I do know that no matter how hard two ciswomen or two cismen go at it, they aren't going to end up pregnant. Trans people, that's a different story, but more on that later. For some queer people, it's really the only option. I hate this word 'option', because it implies that we have a choice. The options are either this, or nothing. This whole option thing also plays into how much it costs and how people are selected for funding.

I don't know about you, but my brain switches off when numbers and science are presented to me, so let's keep this simple. You only need to look at how this book is written to understand how I learn things (scattergun, moi?). So, in the UK, the National Institute for Health and Care Excellence, aka NICE – these acronyms will be the fucking death of me – states that women under forty (who've been trying to conceive for more than two years) should be entitled to three full cycles of IVF. I say 'should be' because not everybody acknowledges this.

And, in some parts of the world, you need to prove that you've tried to have a baby via hetero-sexual sex for at least two years, which all sounds a little *Handmaid's Tale* to me. Like how the fuck are you supposed to prove that – bring home videos and tear-stained pillow cases? What do I know, straight culture is weird. Anyway, the point is that the whole thing is very heterocentric and that being queer isn't part of the conversation.

IVF: Eggcellent if your bank balance, identity and postcode align

In the early 2000s, Guadalupe 'Lupita' Benitez was refused fertility treatment on the account of her sexual orientation. Her local health centre in California claimed that their decision was based on their deeply held religious beliefs (they were conservative Christians).

The doctors were like, 'Oh, we totally want all our patients to feel welcome and accepted, unless you're queer, sorry.'

After eight years of legal battles, the case was settled, somewhat satisfactorily. But Lupita still wasn't happy. When asked why she filed in the first place, she responded, 'People ask me, "Why are you doing this? You already have your kids." Well, I want to make a difference. These doctors are not God. They can't decide who gets to have children and who doesn't.'

Many doctors and healthcare providers do seem to think that they have the right to pick and choose their patients. IVF, after all, was designed for infertile straight couples, not queers. But we all know that the only thing designed for queer people is Hell or Mykonos.

It took until 2016 for the World Health Organization to update the definition of infertility to include same-sex couples and single parents, although the whole 'Where do queer people fit into IVF?' issue is still very much thriving. The system is still designed around those who are *more deserving*. The questions, the language, everything is set up with heterosexuals in mind. And then there's the whole vulnerability thing. The discomfort of queer and trans bodies navigating gynaecological exams, egg retrievals and embryo transfers. These procedures can be extremely invasive. It's like suddenly you're not just the 'other', you're so *other* that you almost start feeling like you've become complicit in the whole messed-up system. Ah, assimilation, every queer person's biggest conflict, the gift that keeps on giving.

And then, there's the dreaded postcode lottery.

Depending on where you live in the UK, the quality and quantity of fertility treatment you'll get can be as random as, well... the lottery. If you live in a more progressive area, you might get access to NHS-funded IVF – not Brighton, though, because apparently the queer capital of the UK is not a progressive area. Tell that to the other fourteen queer parents in my son's school.

Instead, most queer people are expected to navigate their way around a very straight guidebook. We can't prove that we are infertile (because we're also likely not), so we can't get help via the NHS. So obviously we're going to go and pay a ton of money to a private clinic.

As I write this, things are slowly, and I mean *slowly*, getting better for queer people and families in the UK. Like, if progress were measured in… I don't know, Donald Trump-size dicks (first thing I thought of when I thought small). And let's not even talk about the rest of the world, where queer families are still a mythical concept – they either 'don't exist' or are shunned. In many places, queer people still can't even get married, let alone live a life together. So yeah, sometimes I feel like I should just shut up and be grateful that I get to do all the things that straight people take for granted: like getting married, having a family, public displays of affection (yes, I'm into PDA, don't @ me). But then I think, why the fuck should I be grateful for something that so many people just *have*, no questions asked? I know I'm privileged and I'm lucky to live in a place where I can be myself. But I refuse to go around thanking people for *allowing* me to be fully human.

The first bit

Here's a little insight into what happens with reciprocal IVF, and what to expect (although everybody's journey is different, obvs). The person donating the egg (in this case me) immediately becomes the centre of attention, which, for someone like me, was absolutely fine. First, they put you through a full health check, which includes tests, many tests, and hysteroscopy after hysteroscopy until lube is no longer a novelty but an integral part of your week. They also weigh you, measure you… and then tell you that you're actually five foot eight rather than the five foot nine and a HALF that you've been telling people your whole adult life. If anything, that was the hardest part.

Then come the injections. The injections are designed to stimulate the ovaries. I always thought stimulate was a positive thing, you know, a little sexy… Nope, not here. Instead they want your ovaries to produce more than one egg, so instead imagine your ovaries like two bowling balls either side of your uterus.

If you don't like needles then it might be a little difficult for you, because there are many. I didn't mind so much, but I was strangely unable to inject myself, which means I'll never reach my full potential as a failed rock star in the early '90s.

The injections continue for a couple of weeks so not only are your ovaries slowly morphing into oversized watermelons, but you are so pumped full of hormones that it's like that day before your period starts but for two weeks straight. It was here that I found out that hormonal injections and antidepressants don't work well together. You also shouldn't drink, so instead I walked around either laughing hysterically or crying into my non-alcoholic vodka and soda moaning about how nothing will ever be fun ever again. Among all of this are more lube and regular scans to make sure that your ovaries don't burst before egg collection. You also learn about womb linings. Like hair, these can be thick or thin, and like hair, society still finds a way to make you feel bad about it.

The whole time I just kept thinking about the celebrity cyclone in *I'm a Celebrity...* you know, that bit at the end where everyone thinks they have completed the challenge only for the giant balls to come crashing down and annihilate them. In my head, that was my ovaries, swelling up so much that they would explode, sending the eggs flying downstream. But don't worry, that's just my overly insane imagination. You actually have to inject another drug to stop that from happening. Yay, another hormone!

The next bit

When a couple is going through embryo transfer, synching menstrual cycles of the 'egg donor' and the 'surrogate' is a must as it helps create the ideal conditions for the embryo to implant successfully. My ex-wife and I had been synched for years.

For about three years, our periods were like clockwork, same day, or just a couple of days apart. That is, until we actually *wanted* to have a baby, and then, of course, our periods decided to form a union against us because they are bastards like that.

Then comes egg collection day. This is the part most people enjoy because you are either put under anaesthetic or sedation and given a little rest. I didn't enjoy this because I'm a control freak. I had never experienced anaesthetic before, so, of course, I was terrified. I'm not a fan of losing control of my body, which is ironic considering how much alcohol I drink.

Before all this, you are taken to a private room and told to undress. The hospital robe alone serves to manage expectations. I was paying thousands of pounds, and I expected it to wrap me up, whisper sweet nothings and make me an Americano with warm milk on the side. Instead, it felt like it had survived three pandemics and a fire drill.

They then wheel you off into the operating room, where you are given the tea and then told to count backwards. As I said, not being in control is something I fear, but hey, it's 2025, so why not trust a random person to mess with your ovaries while you're unconscious, right?

During the procedure, a needle is inserted through your vagina to retrieve your eggs. I could give you the full clinical rundown, but you're here for the self-deprecating humour and the queer shit, right? And anyway, let's not pretend that I could. But this is where the blastocysts come in.

A blastocyst is the stage when an embryo has grown enough to be ready for implantation into the uterus. This process takes about five days after fertilisation, though sometimes it takes six or even seven days. A blastocyst is made up of over a hundred cells and starts to show signs of differentiating into distinct types of cells. The embryologist then grades the blastocyst based on how well the cells have differentiated and how tightly they're packed together. This determines which embryos are most likely to implant and which should be frozen for later use. Maybe I do know stuff... thanks, Google.

At our house, the word 'blastocyst' became a bit of a joke. You know how when someone gets pregnant, they come up with all sorts of ridiculous names for the baby when they are in the womb?

I'm not going to share all the awful names I have heard over the years in case my friends read this… but you know, things like 'bean', etc.

'Blasto' was our version. That is, until our son was born and we immediately started calling him 'Raisin' because of his wrinkled little face. It eventually got shortened to 'Ray' – which stuck so much that we had it embroidered on his blankets. I HATE MYSELF.

Egg collection is usually a quick and relatively safe procedure, and most people get to go home the same day. When they were done with me, I woke up to the sound of a woman next to me screaming that her period pains were the worst she had ever had. I was warned this could happen. I was then handed an egg sandwich, which I found hilarious but apparently nobody else did.

That night, however, things took a turn. I woke up in what was probably the worst pain I had ever felt in my life. It was like period cramps, but on steroids. I mean, it was bad. I remember being on all fours, sweating like I'd just run a marathon. A couple of painkillers later, and it subsided.

The next day, we went back to the doctor. I told her that I was still in some discomfort, and she asked if she could check it out. I said, 'Sure,' and before I could even process what was happening, she had her arm elbow deep up inside me, feeling around for my ovaries like it was no big deal. I had no idea that a person could feel your ovaries by putting their arm up inside you and having a squeeze, but now I know because I was fisted by the doctor.

The whole process was eye opening, but the most important thing I learnt was how fucking hard it is to get pregnant. Like, there's so much involved: timing, state of mind, your body. I just remember being at school and the teachers basically warning you that you would get pregnant just by looking at someone's dick. But no, apparently, it takes a lot more effort, patience and scheduling. Who knew?

As for sperm! It's not as robust as the teachers at school would have you believe. Honestly, they act like each sperm is as hard as Tyson Fury. Sperm is? Are? It? I never really know how to refer to it. But I'll tell you now, whatever it is, whatever pronoun or verb it uses, it's precious as hell. It only lives for about five days, and millions of them die before they even get close to their destination. They also need the perfect conditions to survive, they are really picky about the weather, and they can't handle stress, alcohol or certain medications. Sounds like every single person in the LGBTQIA+ community to be fair. No shade, I include myself.

The next next bit

While all this is going on, the other person (in this case my ex-wife) is focusing on getting her uterus into shape. This mostly involves drinking less alcohol and doing a bunch of other 'healthy' things like eating carrots, I think.

The eggs are then collected from one person (me), placed in a tube and then taken to the laboratory. There, the egg is either fertilised with sperm (to be then inserted into the uterus) or frozen for later use. A fertility doctor will then select the *best* embryos – because even embryos are judged on their appearance – and get them ready for embryo transfer. The best thing about the embryo transfer is that you get to see it happen – you get to see the conception actually happen, like visibly. This is something heterosexual people often don't get to experience. Not to sound too sentimental, but it was genuinely like watching some sort of miracle. I saw my son from the very beginning, I have pictures of him as just cells swimming around in liquid. Isn't that just *nuts*?

After this, you're supposed to wait two weeks before taking a pregnancy test, though let's be real, nobody does that. Two days later, my ex-wife woke up and declared that she felt pregnant. I told her to stop being ridiculous and wait two weeks like we were told – or at least an hour. But she was adamant, she said she felt odd and that she was going to take a test. And she was right: we took the test, and she was pregnant.

Of course, we were cautious. You have to be with these things, so we didn't tell anyone. But on the way home from work that day, I went ahead and bought three more tests. When I got to the counter, the guy behind it mansplained how to use them. Yes, you read that correctly. He literally gave me a step-by-step guide on using a pregnancy test, unsolicited, and utterly bizarre.

Strangely enough, instead of being my usual feminist self and telling him to stop with the uninvited advice – especially on something as personal as a pregnancy test – I pretended that the tests were for a 'friend', as if I were some awkward teenager. Why are we like this! Oh right, straight culture, but to be fair… they weren't for me.

So, my bit was done, I was obsolete, the focus would soon become entirely on my ex-wife, and it was going to be like that for the next nine months. This was quite difficult because suddenly you go from being very much involved, to being completely ignored, especially when it comes to doctor's appointments, scans, and anything else remotely related to the pregnancy.

But I – we – were incredibly lucky that it worked the first time. I honestly can't stress enough how lucky we were. I had no money for a second try – if it didn't work, there'd be no baby and also no savings. You want to believe money doesn't matter, but it absolutely does when you're a queer person trying to have kids. There's this guilt that creeps in, especially when you start thinking about how much money you're about to 'waste' if it doesn't work. Maybe 'waste' isn't the right word, but it's hard to navigate, especially when there is so much at stake. And that's just one tiny headfuck in a whole basket of them.

Making queer families, one birth certificate at a time

In the UK, the legal status of same-sex parents depends largely on how the child was conceived and, of course, what kind of bullshit bureaucratic hoops you're willing to jump through.

For female couples who conceive at a UK fertility clinic, they are both recognised as joint legal parents from birth. That's right, *both* names go on the birth certificate, like they are *both* the parents or something. The sperm donor is a nobody, a nothing, just a person who spunked into a cup and helped create your wonderful child. He is not listed on the birth certificate and never will be, unless you choose otherwise.

Now, if the child was conceived through that old-fashioned method of heterosexual intercourse with a cis man, the birth mother's female partner wouldn't automatically have parental rights. Even if the cis man and the woman were just pals, or if it was a one-night stand, or if the woman was sexually assaulted. Apparently, the law thinks it's more important to keep things strictly traditional than to recognise the reality of modern families or, you know, rape. In the eyes of the law, consent and the circumstances of the conception are of no relevance whatsoever and what actually matters is that there was a man involved. This sick legal loophole doesn't just insult both the birth mother and her partner, it actively reinforces the archaic and harmful idea that a biological father trumps all other forms of family. I used the verb 'trump' there for a reason.

Since 6 April 2010, same-sex male couples must apply for a parental order from the court if they conceive through surrogacy. After the parental order is granted, both names will be on the birth certificate. To make sure both parents are listed, they can either register the birth together or do a bit of what I like to call paperwork gymnastics/ legal acrobatics.

And for trans and nonbinary parents? No problems whatsoever, right? They should be so lucky. Under the Gender Recognition Act 2004 (GRA), nonbinary genders aren't legally recognised. The GRA only allows you to change the sex recorded on your own birth certificate from male to female or vice versa. So, if you're a trans or nonbinary parent, you can't be accurately listed on your child's birth certificate. In other words, the GRA states that legally transitioning doesn't change your status as 'father' or 'mother' of a child.

The Human Fertilisation and Embryology Act 2008 also makes sure that whoever gives birth is automatically the 'mother' on the birth certificate, regardless of their gender identity. Yes, that means even if the birthing parent is a trans man or nonbinary person, they'll still be listed as 'mother' on the birth certificate. But more on that later.

Did someone say adoption? No, they didn't, but this was all getting a bit serious and depressing and I needed a smoother segue into the next chapter, on adoption!

GAY ADOPTION = DISCRIMINATION AGAINST CHILDREN (ACCORDING TO THE POPE)

In 2013, popular LGBTQIA+ magazine *The Advocate* named Pope Francis 'Person of the Year' – what a great idea, said nobody ever.

When readers questioned the decision, because of course they did, *The Advocate* said:

> Pope Francis is leader of 1.2 billion Roman Catholics all over the world. There are three times as many Catholics in the world than there are citizens in the United States. Like it or not, what he says makes a difference. Sure, we all know Catholics who fudge on the religion's rules about morality. There's a lot of disagreement, about the role of women, about

contraception, and more. But none of that should lead us to underestimate any pope's capacity for persuading hearts and minds in opening to LGBT people, and not only in the U.S. but globally... Pope Francis's stark change in rhetoric from his two predecessors – both who were at one time or another among *The Advocate*'s annual Phobie Awards – makes what he's done in 2013 all the more daring. First there's Pope John Paul II, who gay rights activists protested during a highly publicized visit to the United States in 1987 because of what had become known as the 'Rat Letter' – an unprecedented damning of homosexuality as 'intrinsically evil.' It was written by one of his cardinals, Joseph Ratzinger, who went on to become Pope Benedict XVI. Since 1978, one of those two men had commanded the influence of the Vatican – until this year.

In simpler terms, the Pope is homophobic, but it's OK because he's not as homophobic as his predecessors. Oh, and he's still weird about women.

The Advocate also forgot to mention that in 2010 Jorge Mario Bergoglio (Pope Francis before he was Pope Francis) actively fought against the introduction of same-sex marriage and adoption rights in his home country of Argentina. He then called same-sex adoption a form of discrimination and abuse against children, saying, 'At stake is the identity and survival of the family: father, mother and children. At stake are the lives of many children who will be discriminated against in advance, and deprived of their human development given by a father and a mother and willed by God. At stake is the total rejection of God's law engraved in our heart.'

In my eyes, that kind of behaviour doesn't exactly scream 'person of the year', especially if your readers are queer people. Can you imagine a queer couple knee-deep in a lengthy and stressful adoption process only to see Pope Francis named person of the year on the front of their favourite magazine? It's like the writer of your favourite child-hood fantasy series suddenly revealing themselves as a transphobe, oh wait…

Adoption has been present in human culture for ages. The Romans *loved* adoption but only to increase power and secure a male heir. Daughters were rarely adopted because they only had a womb and that wasn't valuable *at all*. Romans didn't really care about providing orphaned children with stability or a loving home. It just wasn't a very Roman thing to do, like how you'll never see a Trump supporter get a vaccine – it's just not their vibe. Too grounded in reality, too much common sense.

Over the next few centuries, people began adopting 'foundlings', as in abandoned kids who were just… well, found. These little ones could turn up anywhere, and things often got a bit *Wuthering Heights*. One minute, you're rescued from the murky depths of the Liverpool docks, adopted by some random family, and carted off to a crumbling and draughty house on the Yorkshire Moors. Next thing you know, you're falling in love with someone in your new family. Cue a dramatic tale of love, passion and revenge. Can you tell I'm in my Brontë era?

When religion became a thing, religious buildings also became a thing. In England, churches were a popular place for people to abandon their children. Why? Because the Christians kept telling everyone that God would look after them. Spoiler, he doesn't. Unless you believe that he does, and that's OK, you're fine.

At first, the whole abandoning the children at church thing worked wonders. The church would either raise the children in a monastery or nunnery, or palm them off on some family that would then teach them about how Mary was definitely a virgin and how that wasn't strange at all… But soon there were tons of abandoned children, and the Christians needed to figure something out because divine intervention wasn't as effective as a daycare system, hence the arrival of the first Foundling Hospital in London in 1741.

Over in the United States, they had the same problem, but instead of building a Foundling Hospital, they came up with the Orphan Train, which, honestly, might be the most American thing I've ever heard. The Orphan Train moved orphaned children from the city to the country-side, or what was called in those days the middle of fucking nowhere. Around 200,000 children were relocated during its lifetime, which was a whopping seventy-five years.

The twentieth century's two world wars created more orphans all over the world. As a result, the adoption process that we know today began to take shape. There were now legalities involved; children weren't just being put on trains and sent to the country, there were protection laws and background checks on potential families.

But it was still weird. Adoption agencies got all obsessed about putting children with adoptive parents of the same race. Adoption was only available to married (straight) couples because a single woman (single men weren't even considered) wanting to adopt a child was sad and desperate and they should wait in case the perfect man showed up filled to the brim with sperm. I'm not sure if that was what they said, but I'm assuming it was along the same lines.

By the late 1940s, the adoption agencies realised that they had to stop being so fascist about everything and that the most important thing was that a family could provide a safe and loving home. The gays? Hell no! But it did lead to the first trans-racial adoption of an African American child to two white parents. This then opened the doors to international adoption and to Madonna (not the Virgin).

Despite adoption becoming a viable option for many, and agencies continuing to grow, there were still millions of children without homes. Who was going to look after all of these children? It was then that someone, somewhere, suddenly realised that there was a whole demographic out there who wanted to have children but couldn't.

Gays: OMG. Is it our turn? Please say yes! Pleeeeeaaase!!

Lawmakers: K.

()

Same-sex adoption is the adoption of children by a queer person, a same-sex couple or a queer person adopting the child of their partner (step-child adoption).

It took until 1969 for a queer person to adopt (that we know about), but even then, Bill Jones, a single, thirty-something man living in California, had to hide his sexual orientation.

Bill came from a broken home and spent most of his childhood raising his brother. He had always wanted children but had no idea how this would work as a gay man, living alone. He then met with social worker Mary Davidson who told him that 'gay men would make excellent adoptive parents, but if anyone actually told her that he was gay, that her agency would force her to decline such an adoption'.

Bill told nobody, the adoption went through, and he went home with a little boy.

Ten years later, Reverend John Kuiper and his husband became the first gay men in the United States to win the right to adopt together. The Rev had already been granted permanent custody of his thirteen-year-old adopted son because he had hidden his sexuality. But when news got out that the Rev was gay, all hell broke loose (haha, it writes itself!).

In the end, the judge said, 'I saw no reason why this adoption should not be permanent. I'm not trying to get into new avenues, I'm just trying to deal with this one matter before me. I assume some people will be critical, but look at it this way: The man doesn't beat his son, and when you look at all the cases of child abuse you get from so-called straights, you grasp for words.'

The 'so-called straights' burn is curious, but I'm here for the sentiment.

After the adoption, bizarrely the Rev went on to out his son as straight and then went all Ross from *Friends* 'I'm fine...' about it. He then said, 'To tell you the truth, I'm glad he's the way he is for two reasons: one, because it will make it easier for him, and two, because I want grandchildren.'

You know that Math Lady meme – with the equations. That's me right now when I think about this man's thought process: adopted a child but can only conceive of biological grandchildren... Fucking heteronormativity, it'll always get you in the end.

Anyway, despite this minor success story, fostering and adoption agencies were still rejecting applicants purely based on their sexuality. The Children's Society (a children's charity that was originally supported by the Church of England) were revealed to be automatically rejecting applications from lesbian and gay people. You would think that they would have stopped doing that after being found out, right? No. They didn't change the 'policy' for another five years. No shits given.

The queer people who did get approved were able to do so because they were single and could hide their sexuality better. Which is funny, because nothing screams lesbian more than a single woman living alone with her three cats, or is that just me?

That bitch

In 1979, Margaret Thatcher became the first female prime minister of the United Kingdom. You would think, having smashed through the glass ceiling, that she would be sympathetic to the minorities, you know having experienced it herself. But no, she wasn't. She was just a bastard. Can I call Margaret Thatcher a bastard? Yeah, why not.

Thatcher didn't like how her predecessors (the Labour government) had supported LGBTQIA+ issues, so she immediately destroyed everything that they had done. Thatcher's government also became obsessed with gays adopting. I don't know why straight people just love to involve themselves in matters that don't concern them. You don't see me going to Disney World as an adult or being grateful for the sunrise. I don't propose to people on Christmas Day or caption my photos with 'did a thing' or 'mood'. I just leave straight people to it. These are *their* things.

But no, Thatcher's government published a paper about family placement under the Children Act 1989 stating that 'the chosen way of life of some adults may mean that they would not be able to provide a suitable environment for the care and nurture of a child... Equal rights and gay rights policies have no place in fostering services.'

They also encouraged media outlets to agree with them because heaven forbid the media think critically for themselves. The *Sunday Express* wrote that children were 'being handed over to homosexual couples... despite expert advice that youngsters may grow up to become sexually deviant themselves'.

Experts meaning Tory wankers whose wives didn't want to shag them.

The government was just obsessed with the idea that LGBTQIA+ parents were in it for the recruitment. They thought that all queers wanted to do was adopt children and make them gay. It sounds funny, but that is genuinely what they thought, and this was only about forty years ago. They were also obsessed with how queer people would fit into society as parents. If there were two mums, then WHO WAS THE DAD?

Another difficult thing queer people had to face when pursuing adoption was the pressure to conform to heteronormative gender roles, something we still battle with today. Then (and now) the concept of gender role models was massively dictated by the bureaucratic organisation of the adoption and foster care agencies. But believe it or

GAY ADOPTION = DISCRIMINATION AGAINST CHILDREN

not, the sexual orientation of a parent has almost no relevance when it comes to raising a child, unless you are a lesbian and then every single thing you ever do in your life is always related to being a lesbian.

I have no idea how or even why, but many queer people persisted, and some were successful in adopting, but even then, they were required to undergo psychiatric testing (heterosexual applicants obviously didn't have to do this) before a child was placed with them. I've always imagined what went on during these psychiatric tests. In my head, the questions go something like this…

---

1   What lullaby would you sing to your child?
    a. *Twinkle Twinkle Little Star*
    b. *Rock-a-Bye Baby*
    c. *Karma Chameleon*

2   On a scale of 1–10 how much do you want to turn your child gay?
    1 2 3 4 5 6 7 8 9 10

3   Which celebrity do you consider a good role model for you child?
    a. *Ronald Reagan*
    b. *Clint Eastwood*
    c. *Cher*

Then there were concerns that even if they didn't make their children gay, the children would be bullied or have a horrible life because of their set-up at home. On top of having a strained relationship with their weirdo, queer parents. Of course, there was no research on this, it was just plucked from thin air like most Tory bullshit. In fact, we now know that parent–child relationships are typically just as strong in same-sex couples as in heterosexual ones, with research suggesting that gay fathers show greater levels of interaction with their child than other types of parents. God they always have to be the best, don't they!

As you can imagine, this was incredibly damaging to any potential LGBTQIA+ couples, families or individuals who wanted to adopt. It wasn't breaking the law, as such, for a queer person to adopt, but when your government, your media and even your charities are being discriminatory, it just allowed everybody else to do the same. This meant that the agencies were using it as an excuse to discriminate and get away with not choosing people based on their sexuality.

In 1992, the UK government published another adoption-law paper, homing in on how potential adopters would only be chosen if they 'have made a publicly recognised commitment to their relationship' – knowing full well that same-sex marriage was illegal and official recognition of the relationship was hard to come by. The USA were like 'That's a brilliant idea!' and decided to copy it. So, in 1997, New Jersey became the first state to 'allow' same-sex couples to adopt together *but only if they were married*, which was illegal. It's giving *Squid Game* energy.

New Labour, New Adoption Laws?

In 1997, New Labour and Tony Blair came to power in the UK with a bang. The Conservatives were old, dull and out of touch, Blair was 'cool' and dare I say it… not homophobic, to the extent a British heterosexual white man in his forties could be at that time.

In the ten years that Blair was in power, his government introduced civil partnerships, lowered the (homosexual) age of consent from twenty-one to sixteen, lifted a ban on LGB people serving in the armed forces, introduced Employment Equality (Sexual Orientation) Regulations that made it illegal to discriminate against LGB people in the workplace, created and implemented the Gender Recognition Act that allowed trans people to have their true gender recognised in law (a law that has been updated and changed massively), encouraged courts to impose tougher sentences on those who committed homophobic hate crimes, abolished Section 28 (see the next chapter), awarded statutory rights for fertility treatment for lesbians and bi women on the NHS (David Cameron voted against this btw), and in 2002 passed the Adoption and Children Act, allowing same-sex couples to apply for joint adoption (Cameron voted against this too btw).

Sure, New Labour still banged on about marriage and how it was still 'the surest foundation for raising children' but now that same-sex marriage had become legal (kind of), more and more queer people were adopting. They were full and equal legal parents, they could adopt their partner's children, and many families who already had children through other means could now have this legally recognised. Also, in the UK, once an adoption had gone through the court system it could not be reversed. This is still true today. The same doesn't go for the USA, or other countries for that matter.

As of 2025, joint adoption by same-sex couples is allowed in just under forty countries, with many of those countries only permitting adoption if the couple is married. This is difficult, considering that same-sex marriage is only legal in (as of 2025) just under forty countries – though not all the same ones. Some countries allow same-sex couples to adopt but not marry. Why? Because adopting a kid is fine but letting them say 'I do' – well, that's just bonkers. Who knows at this point!

It's also important to recognise that, according to existing data, trans and nonbinary carers are often overlooked. While they *can* adopt and are legally allowed to, most studies and reports focus primarily on same-sex or LGB couples (as well as single parents) without breaking down the statistics by specific gender identities. This lack of inclusion perpetuates the harmful idea that trans and nonbinary individuals either don't exist or are unworthy of being represented in research and data. So, by excluding them from the conversation at the very start, we then reinforce a systemic barrier that further marginalises these communities. Hmmm, where have we seen this before?

... A PRETENDED FAMILY RELATIONSHIP

I'm a lesbian (have I mentioned that?) and I have a child. I had my son with my now ex-wife. He was planned (obvs) and he cost a shit ton of money. But he's not some figment of my imagination. He's as real as the smell of the nappy bag in my kitchen that I keep forgetting to take outside.

The idea that queer families aren't 'real' stems from the infamous Section 28 clause in the UK's Local Government Act 1988, which declared that local authorities 'shall not intentionally promote homosexuality or publish material with the intention of promoting homosexuality' or 'promote the teaching in any maintained school of the acceptability of homosexuality as a pretended family relationship'.

Referring to my son as 'pretend' kills me. The idea of me, as his mother, being meaningless, imaginary, some kind of fabricated fiction, and that he, my flesh and blood, is a figment of my crazed, lesbian-induced imagination, makes me so sad I can't quite figure out how to handle it. Where do you put pain like that? Sometimes, on the bad days, I actually start to believe it. And I wish I didn't, but it sticks with me, clinging like the stench of that forgotten nappy bag in my kitchen. And then when I'm not sad, I'm fucking furious.

The long-lasting damage done by Section 28 is still hanging over us, messing with people's heads even today. So, it's only fair we talk about the people who made it happen, and when I say 'talk' I mean profoundly insult, because if a queer person is good at anything, it's making fun of dickheads.

One day, in 1987, Conservative MP David Wilshire saw a copy of the book *Jenny Lives with Eric and Martin* in a local teachers' resource centre. The book made him mad. Try to picture David Wilshire for a second, imagine what this man, a Conservative MP who gets angry at children's books, looks like. Done? Now Google him. Isn't he just exactly how you imagined him?

This little children's book by Susanne Bösche made David Wilshire so mad that he said, 'the book portrays a child living with two men... [and] clearly shows that as an acceptable family relationship'.

He then enlisted the support of the previously mentioned Dame Jill Knight. Sir Ian McKellen went on to call them the 'ugly sisters' of a political pantomime.

Dame Jill Knight was one of the longest-serving female Tory MPs, which is an achievement, but she shredded her credibility when she started saying that children under two were reading gay and lesbian books. Wait, what children? What books? What kind of genius two-year-old is reading a book? Because I know mine isn't. She regularly threw tantrums that kids were being 'encouraged into homosexuality' and that 'normal families' with a mother and a father were being made obsolete.

But back to David Wilshire, because I feel it's appropriate to really show what this man was like. His greatest hits include, of course, the introduction of Section 28, but also getting caught up in the UK parliamentary-expenses scandal; yes, the one where all those MPs spent our money on things like swimming pools and stairlifts. When asked about it, he said he was 'embarrassed, sad, and sorry' but he also refused to pay it back. He then compared his treatment to that of Holocaust survivors because that's David Wilshire.

Wilshire continued to make life harder for queer people, especially young queer people, his favourite target. In 2000, he voted to prevent teachers from taking steps to stop bullying on the grounds of sexuality. Like, why would you actively want to make young people's lives harder? What kind of person wants to do that? He also (unsurprisingly) voted against queer adoption, marriage equality and the Equality Act. Imagine voting *against* the Equality Act? Again, who does that?

David Wilshire died quite recently. So some may say this is a little below the belt – maybe I should have some respect. But the flip side is libel laws only apply to the living, so… I'm safe.

Take the wording of Section 28, for example. 'Promoting homosexuality' – as if saying the word out loud should be grounds for punishment. This meant that educators were unable to discuss LGBTQIA+ related issues in schools, such as queer families or queer parenting. They were also unable to give students basic and essential information about sex education. Both students and teachers were forced into the closet, terrified of being outed, bullied, losing their jobs. Can you imagine what that does to a person?

I went through all of school under Section 28. And surprise, surprise, my mental health is pretty fucked. Honestly, it's a miracle I'm still standing, because that law was like putting a giant weight on my chest, telling me every day that I wasn't right for society.

When Conservative Party leader David Cameron finally apologised for Section 28 in 2009, Dame Jill Knight wasn't happy and refused to take responsibility. She said it was wrong to apologise and tried to justify her homophobia by saying gay people were 'very good at antiques' – which to this day, I still don't understand. Thank you? Or was she insulting us? What kind of antiques? Does vintage count? Why am *I* not good at antiques? Should I be?

Section 28 created a culture of fear and shame, especially for queer parents who were forced to feel like their families weren't real, somehow pretended. It made people think that queer parents chose to be different, like it was some kind of 'lifestyle choice' and queer families were rejecting the conventional nuclear family on purpose. It gave people a free pass to be dicks. Section 28 basically said that queer families were not real. Discrimination doesn't get more real than that.

But it wasn't just Section 28; the twentieth century has gifted the queer community with a series of defining moments, each one as iconic as a Taylor Swift era. You've got the McCarthy-era witch hunts, Stonewall, the liberation movement, lesbian feminism, 'Don't Ask, Don't Tell', the rise of intersectionality and, of course, AIDS.

AIDS and parents

I never quite know how to write about AIDS without diving straight into a pit of endless rage followed by a deep, existential sadness. Much like with Section 28, we all know what happened. It was shit, but what often gets overlooked in the narrative is how the crisis impacted the growing number of queer people who were already starting families, or the ones who were thinking about it anyway. AIDS didn't just devastate health, it was also a major weapon in the ongoing fight against LGBTQIA+ rights, particularly when it came to parenting.

The spread of AIDS stirred up a tidal wave of fear and hatred, mostly aimed at gay men, bisexuals and trans people. Back then, the idea of queer parenting was still considered so foreign, it was like trying to explain TikTok to a millennial. Look, I don't get it, and I don't want to get it.

Thanks to all the fear-mongering and good old-fashioned homophobia, queer parenting hit a brick wall faster than you can say... hmm, don't ask, don't tell?

But we also need to remember that this isn't just a past problem. It's a very much present problem too. HIV-positive queer people still face discrimination when deciding that they want to become parents. In fact, many queer people with HIV assume that they can't have children. For many, the topic is often ignored or already decided for them. You can't have children, simple as.

Incorrect. Queer people with HIV who are on effective treatment and have an undetectable viral load *can* have children.

Thanks to antiretroviral therapy, HIV transmission to sexual partners is basically a thing of the past. If you're on the right treatment and your viral load is undetectable, the risk is basically as close to zero as my chances of ever dating Yasmin Kara-Hanani from *Industry*. I know that is a niche reference, but I think we'd be really good together.

I can't speak for the rest of the world, but in the UK, sperm washing (which is exactly what it sounds like) has helped hundreds of HIV-positive people create families without passing the virus onto either their child or their partner. Don't you just love science!

And now, as of 2024, people living with HIV can now use their eggs or sperm for fertility treatment. Up until very recently, only opposite-sex couples (with HIV) were allowed fertility treatment, if they ea2tm7merdttawaaéa

K

KIRSTY LOEHR

were in a consenting relationship. But for same-sex couples, if one person had HIV, they were treated differently. For example, when an egg from an HIV-positive woman was transferred to another woman, or when an HIV-positive man donated sperm to someone who wasn't their partner, they were seen as 'donors' and not part of a valid, consenting relationship.

This wasn't just 'simple homophobia'. It treated same-sex couples as second-class citizens, our relationships were seen as not valid, or at least not important enough to be involved in the conversation. It also massively reinforced HIV stigma, which is just as boring as reinforcing homophobia. When are these bigots going to find a new narrative?

b108

AND YOU'RE THE...?

One of those charming little questions that every queer parent loves to hear – in most cases, even before the child is born. I've experienced this kind of shit several times, such as when I was going through IVF, and my ex-wife was continuously referred to as my 'friend'. Then, when my embryo was transferred into her uterus, it was my turn. As her belly grew, I became completely insignificant.

But the worst time this happened was on the day my son was born. He was rushed to the Intensive Care Unit because he couldn't breathe. His other mother had just had a C-section and was taken to recovery. I followed my tiny, barely breathing son to the ICU, heart in my throat, desperately trying to figure out if my son was going to die right there on the spot. And then, just when I thought it couldn't get any worse, I was greeted by a doctor who aggressively asked, 'Who are you?' I froze and said that I was his mum (having only been a mum for about ten minutes). The doctor looked me over again, then said, 'You don't look like you've just given birth.'

There I was, standing in the middle of the ICU, staring at my son who I genuinely thought was about to die, and this doctor had just belittled me in front of every single person in there.

Heteronormativity at its worst

In 2007, Janice Langbehn, her partner Lisa Marie Pond and their kids were all set for a family cruise. But, as they were about to leave, Lisa collapsed and was immediately rushed to hospital. For context they were in Miami, Florida... so you can probably guess where this story is headed.

When Janice and her children arrived at the hospital, they were told that Florida was an 'anti-gay city and state' – ah Florida, the sunshine state where human rights are minimal. This meant that Janice would not be able to see her wife and that their kids would not be able to see their mother. The family were kept away for over eight hours. During this time, Lisa was moved to intensive care where she fell into a coma and died from a brain aneurysm.

After Lisa's death, Janice demanded an apology from the hospital but was unsuccessful. She then sued them, which led to extensive media coverage across the United States. It was this that got the attention of Barack Obama, the US President (in case you know another Barack Obama), who was so appalled at what had happened that he immediately sought to change hospital visitation laws so that patients could choose their visitors. He then invited the family to the White House, where Janice was given the Presidential Citizens Medal, awarded to Americans 'who have performed exemplary deeds of service for their country or fellow citizens'.

Look, it's all well and good that Barack Obama was *appalled* and that hospital visitation rights were changed, and yes, Janice was given a Presidential Citizens Medal. But Lisa died alone, without her partner or her kids by her side. It was completely unnecessary and cruel and didn't need to happen in the first place. But this is the reality that queer people face, day in and day out. It's not just some tragic exception, because apparently being 'too gay to see your partner in hospital' was (and *is* in some American states) the law. So, while it's nice that someone sought to change something, let's not pretend like this hasn't happened since or won't continue to do so.

Let's keep it civil...

On 26 June (my birthday!) 2015 the American Supreme Court required all states to issue marriage licences to same-sex couples and to recognise same-sex marriages that had already been performed in other jurisdictions (domestic partnerships, civil partnerships etc.). As I am half-American (my dad is from the USA) I like to think that this was a personalised birthday present dedicated to me... can you tell that I'm an only child?

A couple of years earlier, in New Hampshire, Marisa and Terrah Pavan were legally married. New Hampshire had legalised civil partnership only a year before and Marisa and Terrah were one of many queer couples to take the plunge.

A few years later, Marisa and Terrah moved to Arkansas. They were in Arkansas when the Supreme Court made same-sex marriage legal across all states. They were still in Arkansas when Terrah gave birth to their daughter. Marisa and Terrah had both planned their daughter's conception, paid for sperm, paid for insemination, and completed the whole process together as a married couple, in Arkansas. Did I mention that they were in Arkansas?

When their daughter was born, Marisa and Terrah listed themselves as parents on the birth certificate. The Arkansas Department of Health did not like this because the state still insisted that marriage meant between a cis man and a cis woman and not between two cis women. So, Marisa's name was swiftly removed from the birth certificate.

The thing is, if Marisa had been an infertile cis man, let's call him Mario, and the baby was conceived using donor sperm, Mario would be listed on the birth certificate as the father. But because Marisa was neither a cis man nor the birth mother, she could not be listed at all.

Marisa and Terrah were absolutely livid, and rightfully so. They accused the Arkansas Department of Health of outright violating the US Supreme Court's ruling on marriage equality, which required all states to treat the marriages of same-sex couples exactly the same as those of heterosexual couples. You know, equality? But apparently, Arkansas didn't like equality.

Luckily, the Supreme Court liked equality (most of the judges anyway – there's *always* one) and agreed with Marisa and Terrah. They ruled that not naming Marisa on the birth certificate was a clear violation of the ruling, since it denied married same-sex couples the same spousal benefits granted to heterosexual married couples. In other words, a victory for equality, and one that also forced Arkansas to acknowledge that, yes, same-sex couples have the same rights as everyone else. Shocking, I know.

It feels like the US Supreme Court's decision to legalise same-sex marriage was like a last-minute 'Oh shit, we're the only Western country that hasn't done this yet. If we don't do this, people are going to think we're weird' – and then when they did allow same-sex marriage, they didn't really understand what came with it, as in, both names on birth certificates, tax benefits and making sure that queer families weren't made to feel less valid than heterosexual ones (maybe that's a step too far).

And you're a what?

We've seen the classic 'And you're the…?' but queer parents also get treated to its equally perplexing cousin, 'And you're a *what*?' – again often before the child is even born.

It wasn't until the 1970s that the US finally began addressing transgender parenting within the context of child custody. While this was a groundbreaking moment in terms of trans representation, acknowledging trans parents and their rights, it didn't always end in the most positive way. I mean, anyone could've predicted that.

One case in particular, in Colorado, involved a parent who, after being granted custody of their kids, transitioned from female to male. After this had happened, they were immediately hauled back into court so the judge could decide whether the parent's transition had somehow ruined their children.

Unsurprisingly, the court couldn't find a single shred of evidence to suggest that the parent was a danger to their children. In fact, their family, friends and even some nosy neighbours said that the kids were happy, healthy and doing well at school, thus proving that a loving, stable home is much more important than whether your parents have a dick or a vagina. Because that's what it always boils down to, doesn't it? The absurd, almost obsessive fascination some people have with other people's genitals.

A decade later, another case arose, this time in Nevada. Suzanne Daly transitioned from male to female in 1983 after her divorce from Nan Daly, with whom she had fathered a child in 1973. Before her transition, Suzanne had been granted visitation rights with her daughter. Suzanne was upfront with her daughter from the start of her transition and, according to Suzanne, her daughter was cool with it (kids are just always so much better at stuff like that). Suzanne then asked her daughter not to tell her mother for fear that Nan would later use it against her in court. Suzanne was right, because of course that's what Nan did!

Nan immediately sought to block Suzanne from seeing their daughter, arguing that Suzanne was now an unfit parent and a potential danger to the child. In Nan's view, Suzanne's decision to live authentically and accept her true identity was somehow more harmful to their daughter than continuing to pretend to be someone she wasn't. Ah, some straight-people logic right there.

Suzanne appealed the decision, but, shocker, she was denied. She then took her case all the way to the Supreme Court of Nevada, but shocker, was denied again because human rights weren't that high on their agenda. Nan then pretended, yes pretended, that she had a court order to stop Suzanne from visiting their daughter. Suzanne didn't believe it, so she showed up anyway, which resulted in Nan calling the cops, because you know, the sight of a loving parent showing up to see their kid was a major threat to public safety.

Meanwhile, amid all the drama (sorry, torment), Nan also had their daughter evaluated by a psychologist. The psychologist noted that the daughter's behaviour had changed, and she had become increasingly anxious. However, the conclusion the psychologist reached was that the behavioural changes were attributed to Suzanne's transition, not the separation, the divorce, and definitely *not* the behaviour of Nan.

At the time, there was no research on how a parent's transition might impact their children. Everything was based purely on assumptions. Suzanne was presumed to be an unfit parent simply because others assumed her gender identity would somehow damage her relationship with her child. There was no evidence to support this, no studies, just a lot of guessing and judgement. Yet, when Nan Daly's mother threatened Suzanne with a gun, that was fine, no danger to the child, no question of unfit parenting, that behaviour was all very reasonable.

Pregnant men

One night in 1601, Austrian soldier Daniel Burghammer (assigned male at birth) gave birth to a baby girl. Turns out, Daniel was intersex. Also turns out that Daniel had cheated on his wife with a man. Fuck's sake, Daniel. We don't know how Daniel felt about his gender or sexuality, but we do know he gave birth and breastfed all while presenting as male. (The Church, however, no longer saw him as an adequate husband – his wife was granted a divorce.)

In 1992, German Karl Holzer gave birth to a baby boy. When Karl was born, he was assigned male despite being born intersex. During interviews, Karl was extremely positive about the whole thing, declaring themself as both mother and father to the baby.

Then, ten years later, Thomas Beatie, from Hawaii, made headlines when he announced that he was pregnant. Thomas's wife was infertile, so the couple had decided to use donated sperm, which was inseminated into Thomas. The couple eventually had two children, a daughter and a son.

Unlike Daniel Burghammer and Karl Holzer, Thomas was a trans man, in that he had transitioned from female to male. Also, unlike Daniel Burghammer and Karl Holzer, Thomas purposefully became pregnant. It was no mistake; it was his intention.

See, there's this persistent narrative that a transgender person is simply 'born in the wrong body' – as if a person's entire identity can be reduced to one simple little catchphrase. But a trans person's journey is not as simple as that, and it's this perceived simplicity that ironically causes so much confusion.

Trans men are frequently told they can't have children, or worse, it's assumed they wouldn't want to. It's as if pregnancy doesn't align with the outdated, arbitrary notion of what it means to be a 'man' – whatever that is supposed to mean anyway. And yes, pregnancy most definitely wreaks havoc with body dysphoria and identity, but that doesn't erase the urge to have children. The longing for parenthood is as human as it gets, and it's not confined to any one gender. People want children, they always have.

In 2004, the UK's Gender Recognition Act finally permitted transgender people to formally change their birth certificates to their identifying gender. However, this did not recognise non-binary identities – it still doesn't. But there is a Nonbinary Parents' Day, which is celebrated on the third Sunday of April each year, honouring nonbinary parents and recognising the diversity of parenting styles and gender identities. So, there is that, in case anybody didn't know.

Anyway, in 2018 trans man Freddy McConnell (who had previously and formally changed his birth certificate to his identifying gender) gave birth to a son. Freddy intentionally chose to stop taking his testosterone so he could get pregnant. When asked why it was so important for him to carry his own child, Freddy replied, 'Straight people don't get asked, "Why didn't you adopt? Why was it so important to be genetic parents?" So why do gay and trans people get asked that?'

Freddy shares his experience in the documentary *Seahorse* (2019). The documentary explores his experience of stopping testosterone replacement therapy, becoming pregnant and having the baby. He talks about the changes in his body during pregnancy. '[Being trans] is not something I can choose, or leave behind, or change. It's not something predicated on my physical state. It's a thing, it's part of me. So if I'm pregnant, it doesn't change me being trans.'

As previously mentioned, in the UK, those who physically give birth are listed as the mother on a child's birth certificate. Freddy was not allowed to be listed as the child's father, despite changing his gender under the Gender Recognition Act of 2004.

It's a rule that makes no sense. An English birth certificate has two spaces for mother and father or for mother and parent. Why can you not be listed as 'father' or just 'parent' if you are the birth parent and legally male? Do only certain letters on the keyboard work? Are only certain letters allowed to take part in this bureaucratic charade?

To make things even more confusing (or actually just fucking stupid) the law states that the word 'mother' is actually genderless. Yes, the word 'mother' is apparently genderless, despite dictionary definitions saying otherwise, along with every single person ever who is dismissive towards trans people and trans rights. It's like they are making up these rules as they go along, or when it suits them.

The president of the Family Division of the High Court also denied a declaration of parentage filed by Freddy McConnell. The president declared that Freddy was legally the child's mother and thus possessed parental responsibility for the child accordingly. Because of this decision, Freddy could not be listed as his child's father on the birth certificate. So, if you give birth to a child in the UK, you will be automatically registered as a mother, even if you are legally male or identify as nonbinary.

But this isn't the same for every country. In Israel, trans man Yuval Topper-Erez gave birth to all three of his children with his husband Matan by his side. The first two of his children were born in Israel, while the third was born in the UK. After the birth of their first son in 2011, the Israeli Interior Ministry initially refused to recognise Yuval as the father (he was registered as the mother) or acknowledge Matan as the biological father of the child.

Yuval and Matan appealed and won. To make the registration work, Yuval first had to be listed as female, so that he could be registered alongside Matan. After that, Yuval's status was changed to male. This was the first time that both members of a same-sex couple in Israel had been listed as a baby's biological parents. In the past, one of the parents was required to adopt the child.

But their time in the UK was frustrating. While pregnant with their third child, Yuval's blood tests were botched because he was still registered as male, which meant nobody looked for pregnancy-related conditions. This resulted in delays. Look, I get it, if someone's registered as male, how would you know they're pregnant? You would be forgiven for not immediately thinking that. But here's the thing, if you actually look at someone's notes, instead of just making assumptions, you'd quickly figure out that, yes, this person is trans, and maybe we should check for, oh, I don't know, pregnancy symptoms – which is ironically what they came here to ask about in the first place.

Now, don't get me wrong, I love the NHS, lots of Brits do. The doctors and nurses aren't the problem. Most of them are smart, well trained and genuinely care about doing better. The issue is that they are not trained in LGBTQIA+ related issues and that there is no money coming from the government to make that happen.

Fertility for trans men and women is barely talked about, under-researched and largely ignored. Trans people are often told hormone treatments will leave them infertile, with horror stories about oes-trogen ruining reproductive systems – all without any real evidence. This scaremongering is not just confusing, it's downright unfair. It has also led to many accidental pregnancies thanks to misinformation about fertility and hormone treatments.

If we had better training for healthcare professionals in supporting LGBTQIA+ families, especially with regard to pregnancy and birth, it could prevent negative experiences, provide better care and stop unnecessary delays. The delays are a massive problem, because there are many. From research and talking to other queer parents, I could write *A Short History of Delays on the Road to Queer Parenthood*, which would actually end up being a long history, but you know what I mean.

Our clinic loved a delay. We would ring them constantly, asking for callbacks, but they never rang back. One time, we had an appointment in-house. There was such a delay that we had to leave halfway through the appointment and do the other half another day (the other half never happened). They also forgot to instruct us on how to inject ourselves, because apparently that's easy and everyone knows how to inject hormones into their stomach. This resulted in us using the final injection on the first day, which then resulted in another delay. But that was mainly because we were stupid. Other delays included a polyp, a dodgy womb lining, some fibroids and, the biggest delay of all, a global pandemic. We also decided to get married, plan the wedding and hand out the invitations with an already booked wedding date. We then learnt maths and figured out that if the IVF worked, the baby would be due on the actual wedding date… The wedding date was changed, and invitations were redesigned and printed again.

In 2012, Trevor MacDonald (no, not that one) founded Birthing and Breast or Chestfeeding Trans People and Allies, bringing attention to the experiences of trans individuals feeding their children in public.

Trevor said, 'I've felt pressured to nurse in bathrooms because of the supposed lewdness of feeding a baby from my body. I'm also told that my body and gender don't fit into the neatly divided men's and women's restrooms of Western society. People like me are told to keep out.'

Honestly, how did we get here? It's mind-blowing to me that someone wanting to feed and nourish their child would be a source of irritation.

Over in Ecuador, trans couple Fernando Machado and Diane Rodriguez made headlines after announcing they were expecting a child. Diane commented, 'There have been other pregnancies of transgender people in other countries [through] in-vitro fertilization or artificial insemination.

I respect everyone's decision to have sons or daughters, [but] in our case it was not necessary to resort to such alternatives as we are able to conceive biologically.'

Of course, the news wasn't taken lightly, because, well, have you been reading this book? But here's the part I don't understand. We've seen people get mad when queer people use IVF, adoption, surrogates, etc. to start families, so why does it also piss them off when a queer person manages to conceive biologically, isn't that what they wanted? Biological, natural, traditional and all those other weaponised words of reproduction. I thought that's what they wanted!

Before I'm about to lose the plot, I want to say this. People need to just *stop* making assumptions! Queer people know themselves better than anyone else, so the sooner people start listening, the better. It's not rocket science. If someone uses the term 'chestfeeding', it's clearly what they prefer to use, so use it when talking to them. I'll never understand a person's need to completely disregard something important to someone else, when it has absolutely no effect on them. The English language is blessed with a lack of gendered nouns, like that's been a thing forever, it isn't new. But also, language is changing, adapting and reflecting the world around us, and it's OK.

Surrogacy: womb service

The modern miracle of reproductive technology has helped turn the dream of parenthood into a reality for queers all over the world. But, while science has blessed us with many options to have children, gay cis men still face a very obvious challenge… someone still has to do the heavy lifting. Wow, gay cis men, the group that benefits *the least* from something. Who would've thought? Joking of course, you know I love my gays, my four best friends are gay men! Although now I just sound like that person who tries to justify their racism by saying they have a Black friend.

Surrogacy has become a popular option for many queer people, especially gay cis men, who are keen on starting families. However, as with anything that strays from that same old, familiar script, it's never without its magical moments of straight confusion. Cue the endless rounds of 'And you're the…?' directed at the dads, the surrogate, and anyone else who might be involved.

In 1999, British couple Tony and Barrie Drewitt-Barlow made history in a way that reflected the chaos of the late 1990s: they became the first same-sex couple to be listed as 'parent one' and 'parent two' on the birth certificate of their twins. The twins were conceived using both Tony's and

Barrie's sperm along with a donor egg from the United States. The twins were then carried via a surrogate because, well, science hasn't quite stretched to cis men carrying babies yet. And to be honest, even if it did, it's not as if anybody is going to tell us about it, are they?

The birth of the twins thrust surrogacy into the limelight, sparking a wave of interest from other gay cis men eager to be biologically linked to their future children. But, of course, as we learnt with IVF, there were legal and ethical battles to contend with, like how some surrogates had been forced to get abortions when babies were found to have birth defects, or if the parents had broken up.

We also have to consider the role of the surrogate. I mean, it wasn't that long ago that Olympic champion diver Tom Daley and husband Dustin Lance Black were accused of exploiting women's bodies after using a surrogate for both of their kids.

Surrogate? More like surro-great!

Here are two different surrogacy options. Commercial surrogacy (compensated surrogacy) is when a surrogate receives compensation (as in womb service) along with all pregnancy-related expenses. Altruistic surrogacy is when the surrogate does not accept payment for carrying the baby, but all pregnancy-related expenses are paid for.

The rules of surrogacy are complicated and difficult to understand. Laws around surrogacy vary from country to country and there also several legal loopholes to be aware of and to jump through. It feels like the whole thing was designed by someone who hates procreation, but maybe that's just me being a pessimist or someone who hates reading legal documents.

In the USA, surprisingly, it's easier to navigate, thanks to the country's unofficial motto 'Everything is for sale' – just ask Elon Musk. Actually, don't. Avoid that man at all costs.

Wombs are no exception, because commercial surrogacy is legal in many states. But seriously, I can't imagine that lasting long. Can you imagine the Trump administration being cool with gay couples using surrogates to create families? You mean, a woman making decisions about what to do with her own body? And getting paid for it? Madness.

Surrogacy in the UK

Surrogacy is legal in the UK, but the 'rules' and legal loopholes are intensely complicated. For starters, surrogacy agreements in the UK don't really mean anything in the eyes of the law. It's basically all about trust. Trust that the surrogate won't have a change of heart halfway through the pregnancy, and trust that the intended parents will pay for pregnancy-related expenses. So, if you're like me, and assume that everyone has an ulterior motive and is out to destroy your life, it might not be the best option for you.

Commercial surrogacy is illegal in the UK, but parents are allowed to pay surrogates 'reasonable' pregnancy-related expenses. In my mind, it's like a lawyer saying, 'Commercial surrogacy is illegal!' but then creepily winking at the same time. There seems to be no clear definition of what 'reasonable' pregnancy-related expenses entail, so I'm guessing a giant brown envelope full of cash is a no, but a couple hundred more on top of a private scan might just be overlooked.

However, it *is* a criminal offence for third parties to be paid for arranging a surrogacy. So, if you're thinking of becoming the Eddie Hearn of the surrogacy world, think again (I don't know how I know who Eddie Hearn is, but the joke felt right). You are also not allowed to organise a surrogacy, take a fee, advertise wombs, or anything remotely Alan Sugar-y (another man whose name I wish wasn't in this book) in that department, unless, of course, you're a non-profit – then that's fine!

Surrogacy treatment in the UK is managed by the Human Fertilisation and Embryology Authority (which we met in the How Do You Like Your Eggs? chapter), which applies a Code of Practice. This code lays out exactly what fertility clinics must do for the surrogate, the intended parents and any donors involved. Mainly, it's a 'sort of protection' in a practice that doesn't really have much legal protection.

Then, when the baby is born, the surrogate is technically the legal mother, and if she's married, her spouse becomes the second parent. This can be quite scary for the intended parents, but don't panic because, all being well, the intended parents will apply for a parental order, which officially makes them the parents, removes the surrogate's (and spouse's) parental responsibilities and issues a new birth certificate. Doesn't this all sound really appealing…

()

As I said in the first chapter, the words 'mother' and 'father' can carry a lot of weight. For many, they mean something specific; for others, they don't really matter. For some, the law unfortunately decides for you. But what's important is that it's your choice.

I remember my ex and I being relentlessly asked how we'd identify to our child.

'What will you be called?'

'Are you going to do cute nicknames?'

These questions irritated me from the very beginning, but I didn't really know why I was annoyed. Was I overreacting? Did I just need to chill out? But they kept coming, all through the pregnancy. It seems that when queer people have kids, there's this expectation to conform to heteronormative norms, and when they don't fit, straight people (because let's face it, they were the ones asking the questions) are desperate for us to fix it, so that they can understand things in a heteronormative context.

In the end, we both felt comfortable with 'Mummy' – no variations, no nicknames. Hilariously, it was quite conventional of us, but it wasn't about conforming, it just felt comfortable and worked for us. And most importantly, it was our choice. But again, this led to more questions.

'How will you know who he's talking to?'

'How will you know who he wants?'

Lucky for me, I didn't have to answer those because we split up, and now when I'm with my son, I'm the only 'Mummy' in the room. Problem solved! But, I mean, you don't *have to* split up. Even when we were together and both going by

'Mummy' it was never an issue for us, we always knew exactly who he was speaking to. Because one of the best things about being queer is that it frees you from those tired clichés. You get to make all the decisions for yourself – how you're addressed being one of them.

WHERE ARE ALL THE QUEER PARENTS?

We've already figured out that queer parents are just as capable of parenting wins and fails as heterosexual parents. We also know that kids of queer parents aren't running around with mental-health issues just because their parents are queer (to be fair, it's the parents who could probably use a session or two – #MentalHealthHumour). So, now that we've cleared that up, where do we stand?

Well, despite there being millions of queer parents and families in the world, their representation in movies, music, TV, and literature is… how do we say this? Practically non-existent. OK, maybe that's a bit dramatic, there's almost nothing. But here are some…

Screen queens

That Certain Summer (1972) was an ABC made-for-television movie about a gay dad (played by Hal Holbrook) who figured out that he was gay after having his kid. Unsurprisingly, it was a struggle for producers and screenwriters Richard Levinson and William Link to get the movie green-lit in the first place, and then they had to cast the main character. Initially, Hal Holbrook turned down the role, not because he was a homophobe, but because it wasn't shocking enough. 'I wasn't worried about whether the character was a gay person or not; the reason I turned it down, frankly, is I read the script and I didn't think much happened in it. I just thought it was kind of tame,' he said.

Tame? All right, Hal, what did you want? Anal beads?

The movie received both positive and negative reviews. It was positive because it was one of the first films to portray a gay dad as nice and not weird. Aww. It was negative because in the film the dad tells his son that being gay is a sickness and that he would choose to be straight if he could. Darn.

On the night that the movie was screened, ABC received a bomb threat. I don't know why this makes me laugh so much because a) it's not funny, but b) straight people can be so ridiculous some-times that I can't help it.

The following year, US documentary *Sandy and Madeleine's Family* was released. You may remember these two from earlier. You know, the ones who met at church, hooked up, left their husbands and moved into adjoining apartments. Yes, them.

The documentary was made to show how happy their children were, which probably infuriated the ex-husbands even more. But don't worry, the husbands didn't sue them again; instead, the court lifted the restrictions on Sandy and Madeleine's living arrangements so they were all allowed to live in one big, giant, gay house.

More lesbian-themed content came in the 1985 US documentary *Choosing Children*. The film looked at six different families (mostly lesbians) as they figured out how to have children. The best thing about it is that each family is very different in terms of race, sexuality, relationship set-up and how they navigate having children. There are donors (both known and unknown), pregnancy and adoption. It's fucking great.

Many queer people at the time had just assumed that they couldn't have children, so to see that it was possible on screen was groundbreaking. Even the director, Debra Chasnoff, was inspired. She said, 'I was like everybody else. I assumed that being gay meant that I was not going to have children. I think the experience of making the film was enormously life-changing for me, because I did end up having children... I think having that possibility [of becoming parents] has changed all of our lives. It used to be when you came out, that topic was off the table. You didn't have to grapple with your partner about whether you were going to have kids or not. It was just not part of your relationship – and now, I think everybody has to have that conversation.'

In 2000, another American documentary, *Our House*, presented interviews with several different queer parents and families detailing everything from homophobia to racism and empowerment. At one point, seventeen-year-old Ry says, 'I've spent my entire life explaining my family to people who just don't get it.'

It's true. Because of the world in which we live, queer parents spend their whole lives explaining their choices. If we're not explaining why we want children, or how we went about making them, we're now having to navigate why we *don't* want children, given we can choose to have them now. I think that offends straight people even more! I've answered thousands of invasive questions about how my child was created, questions that a straight person would never be asked. I welcome the questions because I'm fed up with being othered. I want to normalise the process and make people more aware. But remember, we don't owe straight people anything, we don't owe them an explanation, and if you are a straight person reading this, think about the questions you are asking, where they are coming from, and why you want to know.

The content of this book has mainly been centred around cis men and cis women. But as we all know, that does not encompass all of our community – our community also includes trans people. And, despite the growing community of trans people and trans parents, transgender rights both legally and culturally fall behind in terms of accessible information and how they are represented. I say fall behind, but we all know I mean that trans people are purposefully ignored and vilified by *both* heterosexual and queer communities.

In 2005, the documentary *Transparent* broke ground with its revealing insight into trans parenthood and the challenges and complications that can arise. What's interesting about this particular film is that it focuses on trans men, many of whom transitioned after giving birth. It also provides viewers with information on a subject that is rarely talked about, if not completely ignored, making it all the more important.

It's funny because *Transparent* shows the world how trans parents experience the same old shit that cis parents do – like teen pregnancy, being a single parent, and just how knackering it all is in the first place. But, as we all know, a cis parent's gender is never questioned with regard to how that may affect their relationship with their child. As for trans parents, they still continuously have to justify their parenting in relation to their gender and identity.

The Kids Are All Right, but the film is shit

But it's not just straight people at fault. Nope, members of our community can get it wrong too, even lesbians (I know, shocker!). This one really stings, though…

Written and directed by Lisa Cholodenko, an actual lesbian, *The Kids Are All Right* (2010) was one of the first mainstream Hollywood movies to focus solely on a queer couple with kids. Here's a rundown for those who are lucky enough never to have seen it.

Annette Bening (Nic) and Julianne Moore (Jules) are a married couple living in Los Angeles with their children. The kids decide to seek out their sperm donor, Paul (Mark Ruffalo), some oddball 'bohemian' loser who is supposed to be really cool and likeable. As soon as you see Paul, you know that he's going to fuck things up. He does, and he bangs Julianne Moore.

Jules and Paul end up having an affair, they even fuck in Nic and Jules's bed. The disrespect is REAL. It gets worse, though, because they start playing happy families, in front of Nic, and the whole thing is in such bad taste.

In the end, Paul asks Jules to move in with him, bringing the children with her. Honestly, like, in what world is Julianne Moore's character going to leave her hot, intelligent, amazing wife for this man? Annette Bening's character is an obstetrician!

There are a lot of things I hate about this movie, but what I hate most is how much it champions heteronormativity. It plays into the right-wing 'it's just a lifestyle choice', 'rejecting the nuclear family on purpose' narrative that continuously plagues queer people and their families. Yeah, you can be a lesbian but as soon as Mark Ruffalo comes along, we all know you're going to open your legs.

It's also really uncomfortable viewing. I wasn't a parent when I saw this movie, and I was still under the assumption that I wouldn't become one. This film was supposed to portray a happy, successful queer family, but instead, it confirmed that having children as a queer person was going to be difficult, and even dangerous. No straight parent is under the constant threat that someone, somewhere is going to take their child away from them. Queer parents see this threat all the time, in history books, in the media, in the courtroom, and now even in the cinema – a place that is supposed to offer escapism. No wonder queer people are scared to have kids.

OK, this has been a bit depressing, hasn't it? So here's something nice.

Modern Family first hit screens in 2009 and was a success almost immediately. Around that time, things were (and still are) dire for queer people in the USA, with numerous state laws and baffling federal policies that often prevented queer people from having children.

While queer characters were not uncommon – think *Will and Grace* (1998) – queer parents were. Sure, we had Carol and Susan bossing it in *Friends* (1994), but we barely saw them. Plus, we usually had to put up with Ross being homophobic or freaky about the whole thing. But in *Modern Family*, we had main characters Cam and Mitch, a queer couple, in a settled and loving relationship.

Cam and Mitch are also parents to Lily. Lily originally came from Vietnam, and we see from the very first episode that she has been adopted. We don't hear of Lily's biological mother, there is no threat that Lily will be taken away, and both Cam and Mitch are portrayed like any other parents in a sitcom: neurotic, overbearing, but loving and sweet.

And sidenote, I know we're supposed to encourage queer actors in queer roles, but honestly how actor Eric Stonestreet (Cam) isn't gay in real life blows my tiny little lesbian mind. Give that man a key to the queer city.

Then in 2021, the third series of *Master of None* focused on a Black lesbian navigating the complicated world of IVF. IVF is rarely portrayed in the media, and if it is, it's almost always from a heteronormative and white perspective. Not here. And of course, this woman wasn't just any woman, she was a Black woman, a Black lesbian, which, as we all know, gives her extra levels of complexity that I could never understand.

However, I still massively related to so many things, the hurdles, the loopholes, the struggles of IVF – for example, if a lesbian happens to be swallowed by a whale, there's an actual insurance code for that. But if that same lesbian wants a baby? No insurance code for that – unless she's straight of course.

When you've actually gone through the same thing (IVF, I was never swallowed by a whale) it is so validating to see it played out on-screen. And up until now, I have never seen another television show get IVF so right. If you know of any, please tell me!

I'm at the end of my trope

In 1979, Jane Severance's *When Megan Went Away* became one of the first children's books to portray a real lesbian. I mean, you already had Anne (*of Green Gables*) and Pippi (Longstocking), but apparently they were straight, much to the amusement of queer girls everywhere.

When Megan Went Away is about a little girl called Shannon who is dealing with the separation of her mother and her mother's partner, Megan. Hence the 'going away' part. Shannon is seen wandering through the house and noticing all the missing things that Megan took with her (traumatic much). Both Shannon and her mother are shown to be visibly upset about the break-up.

Jane Severance, an out lesbian, was working at a feminist bookstore in Denver, Colorado at the time. Fed up with the same old children's literature, the lack of queer people but also the lack of representation around parental separation, she decided to write her own children's book. Jane then submitted it to an independent press named Lollipop Power, which makes me hate everything they do just from the name that they chose.

I'm being harsh. Lollipop Power devoted a lot of their time and money to publishing books about gender stereotypes, etc., but then as expected (with a name like that) they also did some batshit things like rewriting large amounts of text without the author's permission and suggesting that the names 'Shannon' and 'Megan' be changed in case people assumed that 'only women with Irish heritage were lesbians' – and that, my friends, is the best joke of the book.

And as you can probably imagine, the book wasn't received well by the masses, but surprisingly, even the lesbians weren't keen. They were all like, 'Well, it's great that you wrote a book about lesbians, but people aren't that bothered by us anymore and we are starting to have children without men, so can you not depict us breaking up and with broken homes?'

There it is, folks, that classic lesbian chip on one's (broad) shoulders. We've always got an issue with something.

Susanne Bösche, author of *Jenny Lives with Eric and Martin*, David Wilshire's favourite bedtime book, wanted to represent the different families that young people have. Interestingly, the book did just fine in its native Denmark, with people accepting it and even applauding it. However, once it made its way over to the United Kingdom in 1983, it was immediately called 'homosexual propaganda' by the media. Ah, the UK, you never fail to disappoint me.

At one point, the book was rumoured to be doing the rounds at schools, with teachers only permitted to show it to their students under 'exceptional circumstances'. As we saw, this then contributed to the Conservatives' infamous passing of Section 28, which prohibited the 'promotion' of homosexuality by local government bodies as well as contributing to the severe mental-health issues that young people of that time still have to deal with today. I've mentioned this clause so many times now, I'm expecting a royalty cheque to arrive any day.

But then came the 1990s. The beginning of this decade brought an advancement in technology, Kurt Cobain, and Lesléa Newman's lesbian parent classic, *Heather Has Two Mommies*.

The book is about a kid called Heather and her two mums, Jane and Kate. Heather gets upset because her pals at school have dads and she doesn't, but then she realises that having two mums is actually pretty great and she's happy again. Which I'm hoping is exactly how the conversation goes when I eventually have it with my son.

Below is an original illustration by Diana Souza from the first edition, which is, incidentally, really, really funny. It's like the epitome of a wholesome, picture-perfect lesbian family – happy kid, nuclear-warfare-hating lesbians, and a cat and dog who are probably named Vita and Virginia.

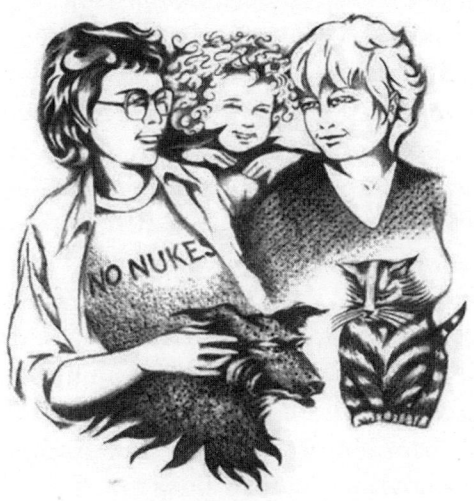

Lesléa wrote the book after being approached by two lesbian parents who asked her to write a children's story about, well, lesbian parents. I'm sure there is more to this story, but the idea that two lesbian parents just randomly approached a random lesbian in the street really makes me laugh, mainly because I believe that it happened.

Again, some lesbians were angry because they didn't think that it accurately portrayed lesbian parenthood. One professor, Jennifer Esposito, said that because Heather gets upset about not having a dad, it gives the impression that having two mums is bad. She also suggested that the book 'dequeers' lesbian households by offering them as 'equivalent' to heterosexual households.

There is a point here, and I believe there is some force to what Esposito is saying, but it's also the early 1990s, homophobia is rife, and lesbians and their children have absolutely nothing else to read, so maybe, Jennifer, just maybe, let this one go.

Professor Esposito wasn't the only one complaining, though: the right-wing lunatics were also unhappy, so the book was banned in some US libraries. But it's OK because it was in good company. Other banned books included Maya Angelou's *I Know Why the Caged Bird Sings* (an Alabama state committee said it encouraged 'bitterness and hatred towards white people'), Margaret Atwood's *The Handmaid's Tale* (for criticising religion... not the rape part, that was fine) and J.K. Rowling's *Harry Potter* series (for promoting witchcraft, *not* transphobia).

Around the same time, Michael Willhoite's *Daddy's Roommate* was published. Is it just me, or do all these books sound like... pornos?

The story follows a young boy, his divorced dad and his dad's boyfriend. This one didn't offend as many people as the others (the patriarchy is scared of lesbians, remember) and it was even awarded a Lambda Literary Award in 1991. But don't worry, there were still some homophobic bellends out there (as always) and the book was removed from a number of schools, libraries and other places where it would have benefited so many different people and families. Heartwarming.

But it's not all picture books and banning, because in 2013, *Radical Relations: Lesbian Mothers, Gay Fathers, and Their Children in the United States since World War II* by Daniel Winunwe Rivers was published.

The book details some of the first known LGBTQIA+ parents in the United States and includes stories of lesbian mothers and gay fathers during the 1950s, lesbian feminist communities, and queer families during the AIDS epidemic. It focuses on how queer families have changed, developed, and dealt with changes in law and new technology. In other words, it's this book but good and without the swearing.

So, sure, there's some stuff out there, and yeah, there's more I haven't mentioned. But let's be real – it's pretty sparse. And when more and more queer people are starting families and participating in society, it can be a lonely place when positive, rewarding representation is non-existent.

THE GAYBY BOOM

The 1980s were a challenging time for queer people. The AIDS epidemic dominated the political agenda, and rightfully so. However, amid this turmoil, queer people started advocating for a wider range of family rights, including housing benefits, medical benefits, social security, inheritance, child custody, and even gay marriage. This then led to the emergence of a new generation of queer parents, giving rise to the first-ever 'gayby' boom. God that expression makes me want to throw up.

The earliest known mention of the term 'gayby' comes in 1990 in a *Newsweek* article titled 'The Future of Gay America' that focused on the growing number of queer people having children. Honestly, could they not come up with something better? The term makes absolutely no sense. A 'baby boom' suggests an increase in babies, while a 'gayby' boom kind of implies the babies themselves are gay… Or is that just me? Either way, it's confusing, and I hate everything about it.

But it wasn't just a shit name, it was also a little condescending. The article begins by commenting on the AIDS crisis and how much focus it took away from other equally important aspects of queer culture and civil rights (because, of course, straight people know exactly how to discuss queer issues without actually, you know… helping).

It then highlighted the age-old argument between separatists and assimilationists. Should queer people live a 'countercultural lifestyle' or 'assimilate into the dominant straight culture' – the equivalent of a straight person's 'Is the Earth flat?' – I'm sorry to every straight person reading this for that joke, but that debate just has a lot of straight energy.

The whole debate of rejecting heteronormativity versus assimilating into the straight world is never-ending. And while there's no right answer, just remember that if you do choose to assimilate into hetero culture, you might eventually find yourself at a gender-reveal party. And if you don't, then enjoy your queer-houseshare-squat, chem-sex party.

The article then goes on to discuss queer families in more detail and how many were lurking among society (in the USA) at the time.

Many are already living the settled-down life of their 'breeder' peers. That includes children — either through adoption, artificial insemination or arrangements between lesbians and gay 'uncles.' There are an estimated 3 million to 5 million lesbian and gay parents who have had children in the context of a heterosexual relationship. But in the San Francisco area alone, at least 1,000 children have been born to gay or lesbian couples in the last five years.

I like how this writer emphasises the word 'breeders', as if they've just discovered that's what gay people call the straights. Actually, maybe they think *they* invented the word, which seems very on-brand for straight culture. Who knows? Either way, it's like someone stumbling across an old joke and acting like they have just invented humour — much like my writing.

What's not so funny, however, is the glaring omission of trans people (as always) and bisexual people, who, let's be honest, probably made up the majority of queer parents back then. Instead, the article stuck to talking about gay men and lesbians, as though that was the full extent of the queer community in the 1990s.

The article also included some examples of 'difficult moments' that children of queer families supposedly faced. Take six-year-old Jacob Rios, who, when asked who the man picking him up from school was, casually said, 'That's my dad's husband.'

Why is *that* a difficult moment? Let me tell you about a *real* difficult moment. A difficult moment is not being able to see your dying wife in the hospital because the law doesn't recognise you as anyone important, being left homeless because the love of your life died and you have zero legal rights, or losing custody of your child, someone you've raised and loved, because you're not the biological parent. *Those* are difficult moments.

And of course, it wouldn't be an article on queer people without the trusted psychologists, because nothing says authentic more than a heteronormative magazine using psychologists to understand homosexuals. I mean, I would've been suspicious if they hadn't.

The psychologists concluded that being raised by queer parents had no impact on children whatsoever, except, of course, for one 'expert' who suggested that they should wait until the children were teenagers to really see the effects. Oh, so you're just going to ignore everything that happens before that, then? Also, teenagers are famously *mental*. Teenagers are mental no matter who raises them. Were these psychologists seriously suggesting that they were going to wait until one of the kids grew up, became a teenager, screamed that life was so unfair – and then immediately put that down to having a gay parent?

It's interesting (and quite ahead of its time) that an article from the 1990s talks about queer parenting so openly, but it's hardly an 'aww, look at these queer people enjoying their human rights' and more a 'what are these weirdos doing now? Madness!' kind of vibe. Plus, the article overlooks nonbinary parents, which is understandable given the era that it was written in when fewer people identified as nonbinary. But now that nonbinary people are more recognised, you would hope that the law would also recognise such societal changes. It doesn't.

As stated previously, in the UK (as of 2025), non-binary people don't exist in British law. Therefore, nonbinary parents are faced with several chal-lenges – like zero resources, no support groups, and, of course, the daily delight of being misgendered. And then there is the lack of data, because appar-ently nonbinary parents are too busy 'not existing' so that it is currently impossible to research or gather data on something that will only continue to become more widespread.

Additionally, it is the same boring, never-ending question that still arises: *do queer parents damage their children?* It seems to be all anyone cares about. The answer is clearly: only as much as the next person! But also, why is nobody asking if we're better parents because we *are* queer? Do queer parents make better parents? Now that's a question worth investigating.

Bring yourself up to the modern day and we have an answer. Well, according to Professor Susan Golombok anyway, and she's a Cambridge Professor Emerita, so she knows everything.

When talking in their *Some Families* podcast to Lotte Jeffs and Stu Oakley (who also wrote a book on queer parenting, by the way), Susan draws on her research from her 2020 book *We Are Family: What Really Matters for Parents and Children* to see how queer parenting can *really* affect our children.

Susan says, 'I think it's because children are not born generally by accident to gay parents, that an awful lot of thought and planning has gone into this. They are raised by parents who really want to have them.'

I mean, she's not wrong. It would have saved me a lot of money if I had just *accidentally* got my ex-wife pregnant, but unfortunately, that wasn't going to happen because it turns out two ciswomen can't conceive a baby… not yet anyway. It's going to happen, though, just you wait…

Susan goes on to say, 'It's not surprising that the parents are very involved, committed, you know, warm, loving, interact a lot with their kids… If maybe couples are not quite so committed to having children, they may fall off along the way. And they may think, well, actually we want to do different things with our lives, and they don't keep going. But those who actually, you know, make it to the end of the adoption process, which is arduous [and] difficult, [and] assisted reproduction can also be arduous and difficult... [So] those who stay caught in there too [i.e. who persist], you know, and do end up having children after all of that [tend to be more committed].'

So, there you have it. We are better. Honestly, is there anything us queer people are not good at?

Anyway, let's move on to something really barbaric from the 1990s, a little thing called the Defense of Marriage Act.

Defenders of the straights (someone has to)

The Defense of Marriage Act, or DOMA (which ironically sounds like a feminist art gallery in San Francisco), was first introduced in 1996 by US Congressman Bob Barr (now the president of the National Rifle Association – of course he is) and Senator Don Nickles. Bob and Don were the North American version of our beloved Section 28 pioneers David Wilshire and Dame Jill Knight. Massive bellends.

The act was set up to define marriage as a union between one man and one woman: 'the word "marriage" means only a legal union between one man and one woman as husband and wife, and the word "spouse" refers only to a person of the opposite sex who is a husband or a wife'.

Everything about this petty little ruling was irritating, starting with the way Americans spell 'defense'.

But also, as if the institution of marriage needed defending. Defending from whom? Well, I'm guessing *us*, but what did they think we were going to do? Make marriage *gayer* than it already is? Have you seen a marriage ceremony? They are as camp as anything. Also, same-sex marriage wasn't even legal back then, and wouldn't be for another ten years. It was essentially defending itself from a threat that didn't even exist, kind of like when Donald Trump told everyone that immigrants were eating people's pets. It wasn't happening, same-sex marriage wasn't a thing. Nobody needed defending.

In fact, President Bill Clinton himself called it 'divisive and unnecessary' – yet still went ahead and signed it into law.

DOMA contributed to all sorts of financial hardships for queer couples with children, such as higher taxes and no tax credits for childcare or education, but it also negatively affected things like military health insurance, base allowances, housing, and even benefits for surviving spouses in the military. And then of course, inheritance and partner protection, which was a huge and detrimental issue during the AIDS crisis.

It wasn't until 2022, yes, 2022, over twenty years after DOMA was signed, before President Joe Biden (who originally voted for it, by the way) finally got around to repealing it. DOMA was then replaced by the Respect for Marriage Act – a much less aggressive term that required the US federal government, along with all fifty states and five territories, to recognise the validity of same-sex marriage and their families.

But it wasn't just DOMA busy dragging queer people and their families back to the Dark Ages. There were other hurdles queer parents were trying to jump over too. Take parental leave, for example, something that was non-existent for queer people, who instead had to rely on annual leave to take time out when having a baby. But there was one shining light, a place where queer parents could not only vent their frustrations but also find comfort in the stories of other queer families. Their very own magazine.

Gay Parent Magazine – a name that doesn't need explaining

In 1998, editor-publisher Angeline Acain broke new ground in the United States when she launched *Gay Parent Magazine*, a magazine about… you get it. Back then, resources for queer parents were practically non-existent and mainstream 'traditional' parenting publications refused to include articles on queer parents despite their growing numbers.

Angeline and her partner Susan were already parents when they launched the magazine, having adopted a daughter a year earlier. Naturally, they wanted to expand their community and, you know, actually connect with other queer parents in the country, their end goal being to include the entire world. God I love an ambitious lesbian.

The first issue featured two gay dads and their adopted son on the cover. How nice is that? But then we find out that during their adoption process, they were subjected to a plethysmograph test (which, just to clarify, records sexual arousal and is usually used on suspected sex offenders). Did straight men adopting children have to go through this? Yes! Oh wait, sorry, let me clean my glasses. Ah. The answer is no.

But it wasn't all bad. Each issue was full of interviews with parents talking about their relationships with their kids and, of course, *how* they became parents in the first place. As mentioned, information was sparse, queer folks were seeing other queer folks creating families but were left wondering, 'How did you do that?', 'Who did you talk to?', 'How much did it cost?', etc.

Fast forward to today, and while we may have instant access to the entire internet, it's still just as confusing. As you have seen from my own journey, there is nothing straightforward or linear about it, most people don't know their options, or, more importantly, their legal rights.

The magazine is still in publication today and remains remarkably popular with queer parents. But, of course, that doesn't mean Angeline has managed to escape the delightful world of criticism. And when I say 'criticism', I mean the pure, unfiltered hatred from people with so little going on in their lives that they actually have time to get angry about this.

This hate came right from the beginning, before social media made it easy to heave garbage from the safety of a screen. Back then, people were a bit more... committed and, to their credit, it's hard to ignore that kind of dedication. Angeline frequently received letters from individuals telling her that they wanted to shoot her. They didn't just type out nasty comments and click 'send'; instead they took the time to write it by hand, locate an envelope, source a stamp and then post it. Nowadays, of course, they just write a message telling her to burn in hell. It's much more efficient for the sender.

Now online only, the magazine continues to serve the queer community, reflecting the world by featuring families of diverse races and backgrounds. It's already challenging enough being a queer parent in a world that still struggles to understand the concept of a queer family, so to have a magazine on your side, showcasing your experiences, is incredibly helpful. Also, by exploring the myriad struggles of queer families of colour, we are shown a whole new level of complexity that white queer parents (like me) will never understand. It's basically regular parenting, but with more hurdles, more unsolicited opinions, and more disgust.

()

In 2009, President Barack Obama made history by mentioning queer parents in a presidential announcement, saying, 'Whether children are raised by two parents, a single parent, grandparents, a same-sex couple, or a guardian, families encourage us to do our best and enable us to accomplish great things.' This was the first time queer parenting had ever been mentioned by a sitting US president.

Obama's shoutout was made on 'Family Day', which I'm assuming is a less racist version of Thanksgiving. And while I'm sure he had good intentions, there was something about his wording that irked me. Why does he say 'parent' when referring to everyone else, but when it comes to us, it's same-sex couples? Are we not parents too? Why does my sexual preference have to become part of the conversation? Why doesn't he stay *straight* parents or straight couples?

I don't know, maybe I'm overthinking it, maybe I'm leaning into the queers-are-too-sensitive or quick-to-anger stereotype. But after years of being 'othered', it's hard not to. Plus I'm getting towards the end of this book and everyone is just irritating the fuck out of me, even Obama.

#QUEER PARENTS

Thankfully, queer families are becoming more mainstream, and visibility is finally catching up with this. When we do see queer families in the public spotlight, it makes our own families feel less like a secret club and more like, well, a real thing. Because it is a real thing, you are real and so is your family.

As we've seen, queer parents are built differently. We sign up for this gig fully aware that we're adding extra challenges to an already impossible task, as if parenting wasn't tough enough. But there are some truly incredible queer parents out there, balancing work, life and parenting like they've got capes under their identifiably queer clothing. And honestly, sometimes just knowing they exist is enough to keep going, especially when you're the only queer parent at parents' evening or the only lesbian shouting at the referee during your son's football match.

Just a few more examples…

In 2022, Carolyn Bertozzi made history as the first (out) LGBTQIA+ parent to win a Nobel Prize. Carolyn was recognised for her work on 'click chemistry', which, despite the name, is not nearly as fabulous as it sounds. I realise this also may have made it sound like I knew what 'click chemistry' was, but *surprise*… I don't.

Carolyn has often spoken about the unimaginable bias and hostility she faced from insecure men in her field, mainly because a) she's a woman, and b) she's a lesbian – two things that send some male scientists into a full-blown panic. But, despite all that, Carolyn didn't just survive, she thrived, even winning a MacArthur Fellowship 'genius grant' – which, according to Ross from *Friends*, is the highest honour known to humankind.

A profile in *Stanford Magazine* after her win reported that Carolyn 'still feels a duty and a desire to be a role model as a lesbian scientist' – and yes, I just *died* at lesbian scientist, I want to be a lesbian scientist. Who *wouldn't* want to be a lesbian scientist? So mindful, so demure, so ready to solve the mysteries of the universe while also probably having a perfectly curated bookshelf.

Also, turns out science *is* the place to be if you're queer, because bisexual father and geneticist Svante Pääbo won a Nobel Prize too, in 2022. Honestly, these people should get a prize for being queer, being a parent *and* getting a Nobel Prize. Like, where do they find the time to do this shit? Writing this book while trying to keep my son alive as a single parent was probably the hardest thing I've done to date. Am I comparing myself to a Nobel Prize-winning scientist? Yes, I am, and maybe this book will earn me one too. Joke, I'm fine with the scathing *Goodreads* reviews.

But anyway, these guys (and the rest) are living proof that queer parents contribute just as much to society as non-queer ones. We are not some rare species, we are next-door neighbours, friends, friends of friends of friends. We are also politicians (not the bad ones, don't count them), artists, teachers, writers, doctors. Basically, we're everywhere, we exist in every corner of life.

Over in the States, they were also falling behind in terms of representation, and it was starting to look a bit embarrassing. So, they made a push to catch up, leading to a surge of queer people being elected to senior positions in a relatively short period.

Kate Brown made history in 2015 by becoming the governor of Colorado. Now, sure, women had held the title of 'governor' before (I love how butch it sounds), but Kate Brown was the first openly bisexual parent to do that. And OK, maybe she didn't exactly end her term with the best approval ratings (she had the lowest of any US governor at the time) but surely that just shows how politicians are always going to be shit, straight or queer.

A few years after Kate Brown, Angie Craig was elected to the US House of Representatives (these American political roles sure have a lot of over-the-top names) and became the first out lesbian parent in Congress at the time. Not long after Angie, Secretary of Transportation Pete Buttigieg (unfortunate name for a gay man) became the first gay parent to become cabinet secretary, and in 2021, Dr Rachel Levine made history by becoming the first openly transgender person (and transgender parent) to be confirmed by the Senate – as assistant secretary for health. Previously, as Pennsylvania's secretary of health, Dr Levine earned national recognition for her leadership during the state's public-health response to the coronavirus pandemic. She also did all that while enduring a barrage of hateful and baseless attacks on her gender identity. Because, you know, saving people's lives just isn't enough.

Then, in 2022, US District Court Judge Alison Nathan was confirmed to the 2nd US Circuit Court of Appeals, making her the first queer parent to become a federal appellate judge (I swear these are made-up positions). Finally, not to be outdone, Karine Jean-Pierre became the first lesbian, the first lesbian mother and the first person of colour to take the role of White House press secretary.

And, as I mentioned in my last book, at this point, someone may say 'Who cares that she was a lesbian, who cares that she was a person of colour? I don't see colour, I see people' – as if that's some kind of revolutionary perspective. And, naturally, I can almost guarantee that the person saying this is a middle-aged straight white man (or woman – yes, they can be awful too, but I prefer to look for untapped lesbian potential in the post-menopausal) who has had everything handed to them on a silver platter, never once having to fight tooth and nail for a position that was historically reserved for people just like them. So, yes, maybe, just maybe, if they had to, they would start seeing colour. Now, let's talk about Jodie Foster. Sorry, I segue using that line quite a lot in conversation.

Jodie Foster met Cydney Bernard in 1993, and the two were together until 2008, during which time they had two sons. To this day, Jodie Foster has never publicly 'come out' even though we all know, and she knows that we all know, and everybody in the industry knows. And yes, everyone has their own perspective on the concept of coming out. And sure, when a celebrity *does* come out, it can help promote diversity and inclusivity, and provide hope to those struggling with their own identities. But does that make it an obligation simply because you're in the public eye? In my view, no. Though I understand why some might feel differently.

Anyway, while Jodie Foster may not have done the whole Ellen 'I'm Gay' magazine-cover thing, she's no stranger to talking about her queer family, often gushing about how amazing they are. She once said, 'I'm so proud of our modern family, our amazing sons, Charlie and Kit, who are my reason to breathe and evolve.'

In fact, Hollywood has a few queer families running around, with Neil Patrick Harris and David Burtka proud parents to twins. The twins, born via surrogate, are basically social-media royalty at this point, and are constantly featured on their parents' posts. When asked about their child-creating process, the couple are often refreshingly open, offering a rare, much-needed glimpse into the world of queer parenting and fertility decisions. Neil Patrick Harris explained, 'We inserted one of my sperm and one of David's sperm into two eggs, hoping they'd both take, because we both wanted to be biological dads. Miraculously, both took.'

Another Hollywood couple, comedian Wanda Sykes and her partner, Alex Niedbalski, met in 2006, and by 2009, they were parents to twins. (Just a heads-up, you don't always get twins, like, it's not some kind of guaranteed package deal.) Wanda, who had previously said she didn't want kids, found herself changing her mind after meeting Alex. Actually, before Alex, Wanda was married to a man and had zero interest in parenthood. So, turns out it took being gay to bring out the desire to procreate.

The couple are very private and rarely talk about their children in interviews. But, you know, that's kind of hard when you're a world-famous comedian. Trust me. However, now and again they will share little insights into their world, with Wanda (a Black woman) often joking that her kids look nothing like her, stating, 'I'm the minority in my own home... Of course, you want the kids to look like you. Why not? You earned it. Go for it. And also, I was like, why do the kids need to look biracial to mirror us? We're two women. We can't make a baby. So their skin colour didn't bother me.'

Indeed, one of the most common concerns for prospective queer parents is the 'non-biological parent' dilemma. It stirs up all sorts of questions about race, genetics, bonding and whether your kid will inherit your eyes or your partner's. Some people really want their child to look like them, and that's totally fine; others couldn't care less. But all feelings are valid, so don't feel guilty for it. There is enough guilt as it is when becoming a parent.

A lot of non-biological parents also worry about where they fit into the family dynamic. It's tough when society doesn't exactly have an instruction manual for your situation. When my ex was pregnant with our son, I found it hard and worried if we'd bond. Even though he's biologically mine (and looks exactly like me), I still had that fear because I didn't grow him, because my heartbeat wasn't the first thing that he'd heard; I was worried that we wouldn't have that connection. It was tricky to find others in a similar situation because, technically, I wasn't the non-biological parent. But I *did* feel excluded from that early process.

But research *does* show that most non-biological parents are shocked at how quickly they bond with their baby and how natural it feels. Who knew you could love something so much while sleep-deprived, covered in shit, and questioning every life choice that led you to this point? Just the other day, my son managed to throw his dinner on the floor, piss himself and then shat in the bath, all within the span of one hour. And for some reason I still adore that little hot mess. But if it doesn't feel like a fairy tale right away, that's OK too. There's help out there, and no problem should fester in silence.

Trust me, you're never truly alone in this and the worst thing you can ever do is keep it locked away.

Jane Lynch (*Best in Show, Glee, The L Word…* how long you got?) is a prime example of a queer parent who suddenly found herself in a 'non-biological' parenting mould. She was married to Lara Embry from 2010 until 2014 and, by default, became a step-parent. Jane later said, 'My greatest pleasure is Haden, my stepdaughter. I'm surprised at how much love you feel and how you would do anything for your children.'

Becoming a step-parent is hard, maybe even harder at times. I know this because I'm dabbling in that area myself. And let me tell you, it feels scarier than when I became a biological parent to my son. At least with your own child, you can blame yourself, or strange genetics. But with a stepchild? Suddenly, you're wondering if they're going to judge you for wearing the same clothes for two days. That actually did happen, and this eight-year-old burned me for it for weeks.

Speaking of blending families, *Sex and the City* actor Cynthia Nixon had her first two children with her ex-husband Danny Mozes in 1996 and 2002. Then, after separating from Mozes, she found love with Christine Marinoni, who became her eventual wife. Christine then gave birth to their son in 2011. Cynthia is not only a queer parent;

she also has a queer child and frequently speaks out in support of her trans son. She's so queer her blood runs rainbow.

Then there's British gay actor Charlie Condou, who made a pact with a female friend that they'd have kids together if they were still single at a certain age. As the big day approached, his friend had recently become single again, whereas Charlie had met his future husband. Not letting that stop them, they decided to go ahead and have a baby anyway. Three adults, three rounds of IVF, and a baby was born. They then went on to have another. Living the dream!

It certainly seems that co-parenting in the LGBTQIA+ community is becoming an increasingly viable option. It makes sense – you get to raise a child together without the hassle of adoption or surrogacy red tape. But of course, it requires a lot of trust. In the UK, a child can only legally have two parents, so if you're a same-sex couple hoping to co-parent with a third (or more) person, it's crucial to clarify everyone's roles upfront. Are you a legal parent? Do you have parental responsibility? Or are you the non-legal parent? For example, if a third person isn't on the birth certificate, they don't have legal rights, but they can apply for parental responsibility.

Queer co-parenting can be a great way to rethink what family and being a 'parent' means. Sure, it's not too dissimilar from splitting custody of your kids after a standard separation, minus the bitterness and trauma of course. But then again, that is exactly why queer parenting works: there won't be any of that, everyone already knows their place.

And of course, here comes the financial benefit. Kids are expensive, especially in queer families, where it can cost a fortune even to get them here in the first place. With multiple incomes in co-parenting, the financial load is spread out, like you might even be able to go on holiday or something.

But let's take it back, back to the early 2000s, when Rosie O'Donnell became one of the first queer people to bring queer parents into the mainstream. Rosie was a prominent, active advocate for LGBTQIA+ adoption rights, often taking on adoption agencies, particularly in Florida (where else!), where adoption rights were denied to gay and lesbian parents. Then, during a 2002 interview with Diane Sawyer on ABC's *Primetime*, Rosie brought national attention to a heartbreaking case involving two gay men in Florida who were about to lose the foster child they had raised because the state wouldn't let them adopt due to its ban on gay and bisexual couples adopting. Rosie was active in support of this case from the get-go.

Rosie has five children, four of whom she shares with her ex-wife, Kelli Carpenter. When they split, Rosie didn't shy away from discussing the break-up, saying, 'I wanted to show people that gay families are just like every other family, and sometimes, divorce happens.'

See, we're just like straight people, give us the same rights! We make the same fucking mistakes! Look at me, for example: my ex and I split up when our son was only two, and we'd been married for a solid seven months. So yeah, queer people are just as capable of messing up as straight people. We're not perfect, and sometimes we don't get it right.

Some people do get it right – comedian Tig Notaro did. She and her wife, fellow comedian Stephanie Allynne (who I desperately want to be best friends with), met on a movie set in 2013. Stephanie had identified as straight until meeting Tig; ah, the power of a funny lesbian, I know it well. They fell in love, married and had twin sons via a surrogate. And here's a fun fact – the twins were born on my birthday, which isn't really a fun fact at all unless you have the same birthday as me, and even then, most people wouldn't be that bothered, would they? But for me, it's great because not only do I have a weird thing about birthdays, but I also feel like this would be helpful in my quest to become best friends with the couple. And while I do have an obsession with birthdays, the same can't be said for star signs – I'm not *that* lesbian.

Though I've heard good things about Cancer and Pisces…

Anyway, in 2024, during an interview, Tig revealed that her son didn't know that she and her wife (their mothers) were gay, saying, 'Their school is six minutes away from our house, and at minute three we were in the front seat of the car talking about something gay, and our son leans forward and says, "You're gay?"'

Worried about whether her kids would be OK with it, Tig asked her son what they thought about their mums being gay, to which he responded, 'I love my family.'

It's a sweet little story, and maybe by sharing it, I'll inch closer to befriending them – perhaps even meeting Sarah Paulson and Holland Taylor. Then I'll have truly made it.

()

We've seen that the law has evolved dramatically in a relatively short time. As a thirty-eight-year-old British lesbian, I've seen a whirlwind of legislative changes in my own country that have worked to protect me and improve my life. These shifts have allowed me to be a parent and given me multiple ways to do so. But how do we know where the law will be in a few years? We always assume we're safe, or we like to think we are, but the future is not exactly guaranteed, especially when you're a queer person, and a queer parent.

We know that queer parents and families aren't going anywhere, and there are more of us than ever. According to Just Like Us, the UK's leading LGBTQIA+ charity, as of 2022 there were around 217,000 same-sex couple families in the UK. This is a remarkable increase from just 16,000 in 1996.

While we might be growing in numbers, there's still plenty of work to do when it comes to visibility and recognition. For instance, the Just Like Us findings report that many queer parents have faced negative comments about their families, and a lot of kids have had to endure remarks about their queer parents. And if you think that's bad, a third of transgender parents reported hearing negative comments about trans people at school. A THIRD.

In a family with two mums or two dads, the parents are constantly coming out, whether it be to their child's doctors, teachers, friends and other parents, while also having to advocate for their child. For me, the findings of the Just Like Us report were both disappointing and concerning as a parent currently in the middle of choosing schools. On top of all the other worries you have when your kid starts school, I also have to worry that my son isn't singled out for having a dyke for a mum.

There is also a glaring shortage of LGBTQIA+ inclusive books in nurseries and schools. I mean, how hard can it be to write one? I've read my son enough terrible children's books to last a lifetime. But I'm guessing it's not a lack of writers, it's more that publishers would rather go with Tom Fletcher from McFly and his endless parade of pooping dinosaurs than, you know, actual real life. The kind of real life where a child could see their family in a book, feel validated at school, and know that their family and experiences are just like everybody else's. But no, let's stick with farting animals.

The lesbian scientist Carolyn Bertozzi (how she will now forever be known) voiced similar concerns when discussing her own family. Carolyn has three sons with her wife, the first being born before California voters approved Proposition 8 (which famously banned same-sex marriage in the state). Carolyn recalls holding her baby, watching anti-gay-marriage adverts on the television and wondering if her parental rights would survive the election.

I mean, can you honestly think of anything worse? Another series of *And Just Like That…* perhaps? But no, seriously, it's shit like this that frightens me every day. In the USA, many same-sex couples are worried their marriages could be challenged or even invalidated, sparking fears about the legal rights of queer parents. As mentioned, in Italy, they're taking non-biological parents off birth certificates; in Russia, they've banned adoption of Russian children by citizens from countries where gender transitioning is legal (this is the same country that bans materials 'promoting' homosexuality), and in Hungary a bookshop was fined thousands of pounds for selling the queer graphic novel *Heartstopper* without closed wrapping.

And yes, while queers are known for, you know, slightly overdramatising – WHO, ME?! – this is real, actual fear. The kind that makes you wonder if the unimaginable could one day come true. But let's not end on that heavy note, because honestly, we all need a little queer joy in our lives, or what's the point? So, let me leave you with this...

In the 1970s, a group of gay dads in Washington, DC started the Gay Fathers group, proving that unnecessarily long group names were just a lesbian thing. Gay Fathers was a space to bond over the shared experience of being gay men with kids from previous heterosexual relationships. The group quickly expanded to other states and eventually morphed into the Gay Fathers Coalition, then the Gay and Lesbian Parents Coalition International.

The Gay and Lesbian Parents Coalition International became the go-to spot for resources, social events, and info on schools, paediatricians and lawyers who weren't trying to take their children away. And, as you can tell by the increasingly wordy name, this is when the lesbians showed up, because why have one word when you can have five, right?

Oh, of course, the absolute best thing to come out of the Gay and Lesbian Parents Coalition International was undoubtedly the children. Why? Because they took it upon themselves to form their very own group, Children of Lesbians and Gays Everywhere. And, because as we know, no movement is complete without a perfectly crafted acronym, this soon became COLAGE.

COLAGE was a place for kids who were often the only ones in their schools or neighbourhoods with queer parents/guardians. It was the one place where they didn't have to explain why their parents weren't sending their food back at restaurants, aggressively playing mini-golf on holiday, or obsessively decorating their bathrooms with nautical themes. You know – classic straight-parent behaviour.

As the group grew, so did their needs. By the 1990s and early 2000s, they realised that the children of the 'gayby boom' (shudder) were, well, a bit different. They were of a different stock. They had parents who had planned for them, using reproductive technology, adoption, fostering or surrogacy. Some were also young people of colour, navigating the difficult layers of intersectionality that come with having queer parents. This led to a refresh in values to reflect and protect these diverse experiences.

Then came the name 'queerspawn', which is honestly a billion times better than 'gayby boom', even if it does give off vampire-tadpole vibes. And also, who doesn't love a good amphibian reference? 'We have queer parents, and we're ready to *evolve* into something fabulous!'

I think that was the campest thing I've ever written.

The queerspawn community has grown into an amazing global network of organisations and individuals who proudly wear the queerspawn label as a badge of honour. They offer support and the opportunity to share experiences. They're not ashamed, they're not broken, they're not the psychological basket cases that old-school psychologists predicted they would become. They're fine. In fact, they're thriving, and they're making sure their fellow queerspawn are doing the same.

So, yeah, the history of queer parenting can be dark, depressing, angsty, and at times so gut-wrenchingly awful it could easily be a Netflix six-part piece of shit (maybe they'll turn this book into a series, and I'll finally get my Pulitzer, Nobel, some kind of prize!). But, for many of us, it's also been the best thing we ever did. I feel this strongly.

Don't let anyone tell you that you can't do something that you absolutely deserve to do. We're just as capable of being parents as straight people, *and* just as capable of succeeding and failing.

Sure, there's still a long road ahead when it comes to things like care, finances and access to resources. But the information is out there, even if it's been buried under layers of bureaucracy, misinformation or, you know, wilful ignorance. People have done it before, and people will keep doing it, because we're queer and queer people are stubborn like that.

And hey, if you don't want kids, that's perfectly fine too. After everything I've written, researched and painfully presented to you, I want to end this book by telling you it's actually OK not to want kids at all. I mean, that's the beauty of being human: choices. We have choices, people! The kind of choices that let us mess up our lives in a variety of ways and then pick the one that suits us best. Want children? Go for it. Don't want children? Enjoy weekend mornings! Want to adopt a cat instead? Live your truth. I mean, you could always do what I did, adopt two senior cats, then a kitten, have a baby, get married, and then separate seven months later, all in a one-bedroom flat. Not chaotic in the slightest.

POSTSCRIPT

Just when I thought this book was finished, and ready to hit the shelves, the UK Supreme Court ruled that under the Equality Act 2010, 'sex' now officially means *biological sex as recorded at birth.*

In response to the decision, Prime Minister Keir Starmer said, 'A woman is an adult human female' – because there's no one more qualified to define womanhood than a straight cisman. Funny, that, because back in 2022, Keir Starmer said, 'A woman is a female adult, and in addition to that, trans women are women — and that is not just my view, that is actually the law.'

One might assume he was pandering to the queer community for votes. And one would be absolutely correct.

The ruling makes it even harder for trans parents to be recognised as 'mother,' 'father,' or even just 'parent' in a way that reflects their actual identity. Legal forms at schools, clinics, or courts will likely default to birth sex, cue the deadnaming, the othering, and everything else that makes trans parents feel like they are invisible.

More than anything, though, this ruling is a reminder of how fragile queer legal rights really are. I started this book in 2023, finished it in 2025, and already some of it reads like a time capsule. It's exhausting. It's unpredictable. And it's unfair to expect queer people, especially queer parents, to live with our rights dangling by a thread, constantly one court case away from being erased.

ACKNOWLEDGEMENTS

Huge thanks to Oneworld Publications, and especially my editor, Cecilia Stein. You've given me yet another chance to write about queer people doing cool stuff, and I'll always be so grateful. I also deeply appreciate your patience with my late-night, chaotic emails (many of which didn't even have a subject line), particularly when I questioned myself. Your calm, reassuring responses were exactly what I needed.

Thank you to Hammy, Mum, Dad, Bash (Lorbes, Tam Pyow, Fox, JW), Kitchen Club, Ericka, and exes with children, for the continued laughs and support. Thanks to Uncle Sam and Uncle Callum (as you are now referred to) for being incredible friends but, more importantly, great role models and mentors to my son. One of my favourite parts of motherhood is watching him connect with you both and see you as I did when we first formed our own friendships.

Writing this book while working full time and raising my son alone was a struggle. There were moments when I didn't think I could do it, when the research was triggering and overwhelming. There were times I couldn't talk about the book with anyone because it stressed me out – sorry, Callum. But there were also moments of laughter, gratitude, and awe for the history that made it possible for me to experience parenthood and to forever share my days with my favourite person in the world. Thank you to all the queer parents and families out there.

Oh, and of course, not forgetting my very own 'Mrs Dalloway' – you have helped me more than anybody, thanks for being… well, just you.

A NOTE ON SOURCES

For a more serious account of queer parenting, check out *Sapphistries: A Global History of Love Between Women* by Leila J. Rupp (New York University Press, 2009). Some other great sources include *The Lesbian History Sourcebook: Love and Sex Between Women in Britain from 1780 to 1970* by Alison Oram and Annmarie Turnbull (Routledge, 2001) and *The Queer Parent* by Lotte Jeffs and Stu Oakley (Bluebird, 2023). Lotte Jeffs and Stu Oakley also present the parenting podcast, *From Gay to Ze*. Nigel Nicolson wrote a great personal memoir of his parents, Vita Sackville-West and Harold Nicolson: *Portrait of a Marriage* (Weidenfeld & Nicolson, 1973).

Further sources include *The Complete Letters of Oscar Wilde* (Henry Holt and Co., 2000), *Different Daughters: A History of the Daughters of Bilitis and the Rise of the Lesbian Rights Movement* by Marcia M. Gallo (Seal Press, 2007), *Radical Relations: Lesbian Mothers, Gay Fathers, and Their Children in the United States since World War II* by Daniel Winunwe Rivers (The University of North Carolina Press, 2015), *Queer Conception: The Complete Fertility Guide for Queer and Trans Parents-to-Be* by Kristin Kali (Sasquatch Books, 2022), *Sperm Not Included: The Queer Couple's Guide to Getting Pregnant in the UK* by Sarah Wayne (Love and Science UK, 2024), *Outrageous!: The Story of Section 28 and Britain's Battle for LGBT Education* by Paul Baker (Reaktion Books, 2023), *When Megan Went Away* by Jane Severance (Lollipop Power, 1979), *Heather Has Two Mommies* by Lesléa Newman (Alyson Books, 1989) and *Daddy's Roommate* by Michael Willhoite (Alyson Books, 1990).

For film, we have documentaries: *Sandy and Madeleine's Family* (1973), *In the Best Interests of the Children* (1977), *Choosing Children* (1985), *Seahorse* (2019), *Our House* (2000), *Transparent* (2005); movies: *That Certain Summer* (1972), *The Kids Are All Right* (2010); and TV shows: *Modern Family* (2009–20) and *Master of None* (2015–21).